Fetal Monitoring and Assessment

Susan Martin Tucker, MSN, RN, PHN, CNAA
Nursing and Health Care Consultant
Quality Management and Perinatal Systems
Windsor, California

FIFTH EDITION

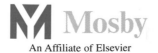

Mosby
An Affiliate of Elsevier

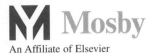
An Affiliate of Elsevier

11830 Westline Industrial Drive
St. Louis, Missouri 63146

POCKET GUIDE TO FETAL MONITORING AND ASSESSMENT,
FIFTH EDITION

Notice

Nursing is an ever-changing field. Standard safety precautions must be
followed, but as new research and clinical experience broaden our
knowledge, changes in treatment and drug therapy may become
necessary or appropriate. Readers are advised to check the most current
product information provided by the manufacturer of each drug to be
administered to verify the recommended dose, the method and duration
of administration, and contraindications. It is the responsibility of the
licensed prescriber, relying on experience and knowledge of the patient,
to determine dosages and the best treatment for each individual patient.
Neither the publisher nor the author assumes any liability for any injury
and/or damage to persons or property arising from this publication.

Previous editions copyrighted 1988, 1992, 1996, and 2000

ISBN-13: 978-0-323-02606-2
ISBN-10: 0-323-02606-0

Executive Editor: Michael S. Ledbetter
Senior Developmental Editor: Laurie K. Gower
Publishing Services Manager: John Rogers
Senior Project Manager: Beth Hayes
Design Manager: Gail Morey Hudson
Cover photograph: Courtesy Lennart Nilsson/Albert Bonniers Förlag AB,
A Child is Born, Dell Publishing Company

Printed in United States of America

Last digit is the print number: 9 8 7 6 5 4 3 2

Assistant Editor

Dodi Gauthier, MEd, RNC
Coordinator, Perinatal Outreach and Maternal Transport
Cottage Health System
Santa Barbara, California

Contributors

Meichelle Arntz, BSN, RNC, ACCE
Perinatal Nurse
Instructor, Santa Barbara City College
Santa Barbara, California

Lisa Berry, MSN, RNC
Staff Nurse, Labor and Delivery
Presbyterian Intercommunity Hospital
Whittier, California

Linda Goodwin, MEd, RNC
Coordinator, Quality Improvement
Evergreen Healthcare
Kirkland, Washington

Evelyn M. Hom, MS, RN, CNS
Perinatal Clinical Specialist
Tacoma General Hospital
Tacoma, Washington

Patricia Robin McCartney, PhD, RNC, FAAN
Clinical Professor, School of Nursing
The State University of New York
Staff Nurse, Labor and Delivery
Sisters of Charity Hospital
Buffalo, New York

Consultants

Julie M.R. Arafeh, MSN, RN
Perinatal Outreach Coordinator/Educator
Stanford University
Palo Alto, California

Bonnie Flood Chez, MSN, RNC
President
Nursing Education Resources, Inc.
Tampa, Florida

M. Cecile Graf, MSN, RNC, CNS
Clinical Nurse Specialist, High Risk Obstetrics
Nebraska Methodist Hospital
Bellevue, Nebraska

Carole J. Harvey, MS, RNC
Clinical Nurse Specialist, High Risk Obstetrics
Northside Hospital
Atlanta, Georgia

Julie Holden, BSN, RNC
Clinical Nurse Manager
Saints Memorial Medical Center
Lowell, Massachusetts

Laura R. Mahlmeister, PhD, RN
President, Mahlmeister & Associates
Staff Nurse
The Birth Center at San Francisco General Hospital
Clinical Professor
University of California
San Francisco, California

Martina L. Porter, MS, MBA, RNC
Principal and Consultant
The Letko Porter Group
Alexandria, Virginia

Catherine Rommal, MBA, RNC, CPHRM, FASHRM
Principal and Consultant
Perinatal Risk Consulting
Big Bear Lake, California

Barry Schifrin, MD, FACOG
Clinical Professor of Obstetrics and Gynecology
Loma Linda School of Medicine
Formerly, Director of OB/Gyn Residency Program
Glendale Adventist Medical Center
Glendale, California

Barbara S. Tewell, BSN, RNC
Perinatal Staff Nurse
University of Utah Hospital and Clinics
Salt Lake Regional Medical Center
Salt Lake City, Utah

Acknowledgments

GE Medical Systems Information Technologies
Milwaukee, Wisconsin

Hill-Rom Company, Inc.
Batesville, Indiana

Nellcor Puritan Bennett, Inc.
Pleasanton, California

Philips Medical Systems
Böblingen, Germany

Preface

Welcome to *the* most practical and portable book on fetal monitoring and assessment. The purpose of the fifth edition of *Fetal Monitoring and Assessment* is to provide the most practical and portable, state-of-the-art information on fetal monitoring and assessment in the antepartum and intrapartum periods. Updated with the most current information, this edition provides a single source of readily accessible information on fetal heart rate monitoring as well as other methods of fetal surveillance. This thoroughly revised edition is intended to promote the evidence-based practice of the clinician who assesses the fetal/maternal patient, identifies and interprets data, and intervenes to promote high-quality outcomes.

Description

This book presents the application of current theory and practice of antepartum and intrapartum fetal monitoring and assessment in the clinical environment. Information is provided about the relationship between acute intrapartum events and cerebral palsy; the physiological basis for monitoring, auscultation, instrumentation, and application of the electronic fetal monitor; computer-based analysis and archival systems; identification and interpretation of data; adjunct methods of assessment (including fetal pulse oximetry); interventions for nonreassuring fetal status; influence of gestational age on fetal data; fetal evaluation in the presence of maternal trauma; patient care; and risk management in the perinatal setting.

Features

Some of the unique features of this book are as follows:
- Content follows a logical and progressive sequence with *advanced* concepts to augment the information base for the experienced clinician and *basic* elements to provide the

foundation in fetal monitoring for those who are new to the subject matter.

- The liberal use of tables, charts, and graphs makes it easier to locate and access key information, such as the sequence of physiological processes that produce decelerations, interpretation of fetal heart rate patterns, and interventions for nonreassuring patterns.
- Multiple monitor strips and other figures are included for their educational value to support and supplement the content.
- A consistent format provides definitions, descriptions, characteristics, etiologies, clinical significance, and interventions for fetal heart rate patterns.
- Procedures are written in a step-by-step format and include their rationales.

Organization

Chapter 1 provides an overview of fetal monitoring. It includes information on the comparability of neonatal outcomes when the fetal heart rate is assessed by intermittent auscultation and by electronic fetal monitoring, and it lists the *new criteria* that define an acute intrapartum hypoxic event sufficient to cause permanent neurological impairment such as cerebral palsy.

Chapter 2 discusses the physiological basis for monitoring. Characteristic fetal heart rate patterns result from hypoxic and nonhypoxic stresses or stimulation. This chapter describes the factors involved in fetal oxygenation including uterofetoplacental circulation and physiology of fetal heart rate regulation. In addition, a list of maternal and fetal risk factors is included to better identify those patients who may be at risk for uteroplacental insufficiency.

Chapter 3 covers instrumentation for both auscultation and electronic fetal monitoring and provides step-by-step procedures with rationales for the application of monitoring devices. Also presented are artifact detection, troubleshooting the monitor, telemetry with waterproof transducers (for patients in bed, ambulating, or in the bath), computer-based systems (with central stations, analysis/alert capability, and data storage), considerations related to monitor purchase, and patient and family education.

Chapter 4 presents information on uterine activity palpation and electronic monitoring with a discussion of normal uterine activity, dysfunctional or abnormal labor patterns, and increased uterine activity with interventions.

Chapter 5 provides definitions, descriptions/characteristics, etiology, clinical significance, and interventions for fetal heart rate patterns that are demonstrated by actual tracings. Definitions are based on those of the National Institute of Child Health and Human Development. Much of the content is provided in an outline format with several tables for instant access to information. A table summarizes the identification and management of each specific pattern.

Chapter 6 presents and contrasts reassuring and nonreassuring patterns, and it lists specific interventions and related rationales for nonreassuring fetal status. A handy checklist for assessing the fetal heart rate and uterine activity is provided for the rapid interpretation of tracings. A *new* management protocol is included for the use of fetal pulse oximetry as an adjunct to FHR monitoring.

Chapter 7 is *new* in this edition and discusses the influence of gestational age on the interpretation of fetal heart rate. The preterm fetus and the postterm fetus have characteristic heart rate patterns as a result of maturational factors and behavioral states that must be considered during both antepartum and intrapartum monitoring.

Chapter 8, also *new* in this edition, presents options for performing fetal assessment in the nonobstetrical setting—for example, during transport, when associated with trauma, emergency services, and during nonobstetrical surgical procedures. A sample triage tool is provided for managing the pregnant patient in the emergency department, and a decision tree is provided for managing the unstable pregnant trauma victim. In addition, physiological adaptations to pregnancy are listed to avoid their being interpreted as pathological, which they indeed might be in the nonpregnant woman.

Chapter 9 presents biophysical and biochemical methods of antepartum testing, including the nonstress test, the contraction stress test, vibroacoustic stimulation, ultrasound, the biophysical profile, an algorithm for antepartum testing, and fetal lung maturity tests.

Chapter 10 provides guidelines for care of the monitored patient from the time of admission through the stages of labor and the immediate postpartum period. In addition, guidelines for documentation are included to ensure a complete and accurate medical record, whether it is computer based or on paper.

Chapter 11, on risk management, has much *new* information on human error, common errors in perinatal units, characteristics of high-reliability units, practical and readily applicable guidelines for promoting safety and decreasing exposure to risk, management of risks and adverse outcomes, elements of malpractice, chain of command, and reporting of sentinel events in the perinatal setting.

The Appendix is provided for colleagues outside of North America who monitor patients at a paper speed of 1 cm/min, as contrasted with the faster 3-cm/min speed used primarily in North America.

Fetal Monitoring and Assessment is intended to be used by professional registered nurses, nurse midwives, medical students, physicians, clinical specialists, educators, and risk management and medical-legal professionals who have a theoretical background in obstetrics. In addition, the format provides essential concepts in a clear, concise, and easily understandable manner for those who are new to fetal monitoring/cardiotocograpy.

The author expresses gratitude, as always, to Larry Tucker for his support of yet another edition, and acknowledges the roles of daughters Karrie Tucker Stewart and Jill Marie Tucker, who were the original impetuses for the creation of this book, and of grandchildren Lauren, Kyle, and Erika Stewart, the stimuli for (and rewards of) the revisions.

Susan Martin Tucker

Contents

Overview of Fetal Monitoring

1

Relationship Between Hypoxia and Cerebral Palsy

Electronic fetal monitoring (EFM) was developed to reduce infant mortality and morbidity. In 2000, EFM continued to be the most prevalent obstetrical procedure, used in 84% of live births in the United States, whereas ultrasound imaging was used in 67% of live births (CDC, 2002). EFM was intended to screen for intrapartum asphyxia severe enough to cause neurological damage, including cerebral palsy, so that timely intervention would prevent injury or death. However, meta-analyses of clinical trials have failed to demonstrate improved infant morbidity or mortality with EFM compared with intermittent auscultation (IA) of the fetal heart rate (FHR). There has never been a clinical trial comparing neonatal outcomes with EFM or IA and a control of no FHR assessment; and for ethical reasons such a trial would be unlikely.

The incidence of cerebral palsy has remained unchanged since the inception of electronic fetal monitoring. New understandings about the causes of cerebral palsy and neonatal encephalopathy have been reported. "A Template for Defining a Causal Relation Between Acute Intrapartum Events and Cerebral Palsy: International Consensus Statement," was published by MacLennan in 1999 and has been endorsed by many obstetrical and pediatric societies around the world. More recently, a monograph entitled "Neonatal Encephalopathy and Cerebral Palsy: Defining the Pathogenesis and Physiology" was published in 2003 by the American College of Obstetricians and Gynecologists and the American Academy of Pediatrics (Hankins, Speer, 2003). These reports define cerebral palsy, neonatal encephalopathy, and acute intrapartum hypoxia, also termed hypoxic–ischemic encephalopathy (HIE), and list the clinical findings that link hypoxia and cerebral palsy.

Acute intrapartum hypoxia, also termed hypoxic–ischemic encephalopathy (HIE), is infrequently the cause of neonatal encephalopathy and cerebral palsy. HIE comprises a small subset of conditions that cause neonatal encephalopathy, and neonatal encephalopathy comprises a small subset of conditions that cause cerebral palsy (Figure 1-1). The incidence of neonatal encephalopathy attributed to acute intrapartum hypoxia is 1.6 per 10,000 births (Badawi et al, 1998). For cerebral palsy to be attributed to HIE, there must be evidence of neonatal encephalopathy having occurred as well (ACOG, AAP, 2003).

Recent studies indicate that, in most cases, the events and conditions leading to neonatal encephalopathy and cerebral palsy occur in the fetus before labor or in the newborn after delivery, and not during the intrapartum period. These events and conditions include prematurity, intrauterine growth restriction, genetic or early developmental causes, fetal infection, coagulation and autoimmune disorders, and trauma (Freeman et al, 2003). These events and conditions should be considered when applying the criteria before an intrapartum hypoxic cause of cerebral palsy can be considered.

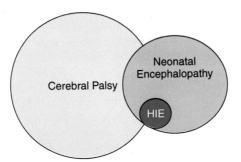

Figure 1-1
Relationship of hypoxic–ischemic encephalopathy (HIE), also known as acute intrapartum hypoxia, to neonatal encephalopathy and cerebral palsy. NOTE: HIE is a small subset of conditions that cause neonatal encephalopathy, which is a subset of conditions that cause cerebral palsy.
(Courtesy Dr. Patricia McCartney, Buffalo, N.Y.)

Criteria That Define an Acute Intrapartum Hypoxic Event Sufficient to Cause Permanent Neurological Impairment*

Essential criteria

All of the following four criteria must be met (Hankins, Speer, 2003).

1. Evidence of a metabolic acidosis in intrapartum fetal, umbilical arterial cord, or very early neonatal blood sample obtained at delivery (pH <7.00 and base deficit >12 mmol/L)
2. Early onset of severe or moderate neonatal encephalopathy in infants of ≥34 weeks' gestation
3. Cerebral palsy of the spastic quadriplegic or dyskinetic type
4. Exclusion of other identifiable etiologies, such as trauma, coagulation disorders, infectious conditions, or genetic disorders (Hankins, Speer, 2003)

Criteria that together suggest an intrapartum timing but apart are nonspecific

1. A sentinel (signal) hypoxic event occurring immediately before or during labor
2. A sudden, rapid, and sustained deterioration of the fetal heart rate pattern (fetal bradycardia, or the absence of FHR variability in the presence of persistent late or variable decelerations [NICHD, 1997; Hankins, Speer, 2003]), usually after the hypoxic sentinel event, when the pattern was previously normal
3. Apgar scores of 0-3 for longer than 5 minutes
4. Early evidence of multisystem involvement within 72 hours of birth (Hankins, Speer, 2003)
5. Early imaging evidence of acute cerebral abnormality

There are several subtypes of cerebral palsy, but the only ones associated with acute hypoxic intrapartum events are spastic quadriplegia and, less commonly, dyskinetic cerebral palsy. Spastic quadriplegia, however, is not specific to intrapartum hypoxia and is caused by other factors as well. For cerebral palsy to be attributed to an acute intrapartum hypoxic insult, there must also be evidence of neonatal encephalopathy. This is usually demonstrated by abnormalities of behavior of moderate severity (e.g., respiratory

*Adapted from MacLennan, 1999.

difficulties, depressed tone and reflexes, seizures) within the early neonatal period for neonates of more than 34 weeks' gestation and often within 24 hours of delivery. Except for seizure activity, it is more difficult to define neonatal encephalopathy in infants of less than 34 weeks' gestation (MacLennan, 1999).

Fetal heart rate patterns that are "predictive of current or impending fetal asphyxia of such severity that the fetus is at risk of neurological and other fetal damage or death" were identified by the Research Planning Workshop on Fetal Monitoring of the National Institute of Child Health and Development (NICHD) in 1997 (p. 1389). These patterns include the following:

1. Recurrent late decelerations with absent fetal heart rate (FHR) variability
2. Variable decelerations with absent FHR variability
3. Substantial bradycardia with absent FHR variability

In addition, the NICHD group agreed that FHR tracings with all of the following characteristics confer an extremely high predictability of a normally oxygenated fetus.

1. Normal baseline rate
2. Normal (moderate) FHR variability
3. Presence of FHR accelerations
4. Absence of FHR decelerations

The standardized definitions to guide research in electronic fetal heart rate monitoring published by the National Institute of Child Health and Human Development (NICHD, 1997) were developed by an expert panel and have contributed to consistency in terminology and definitions. Before this publication, there was a major multidisciplinary impediment to progress in EFM practice, education, and research because of the lack of agreement on definitions of EFM tracing characteristics and on interpretations of tracings. Research shows that clinicians agree on interpretation when an EFM tracing is reassuring yet disagree when a tracing is nonreassuring. In many cases, the fetus with a nonreassuring tracing is often healthy at birth, demonstrating a high rate of false-positive findings. Adjunct fetal assessment methods provide additional information for evaluating fetal status in the presence of nonreassuring tracings.

Historical Overview

Although fetal heart tones were first heard in the seventeenth century, clinician assessment and description of the FHR began in the early nineteenth century with unassisted auscultation (ear-to-abdomen) and later included auscultation with a stethoscope. In 1917, the head stethoscope, or DeLee-Hillis fetoscope, was first reported in the literature. During the 1950s, physicians, including Edward Hon in the United States, Caldeyro-Barcia in Uruguay, and Hammacher in Germany, developed electronic devices to continuously measure and record the FHR and uterine activity. The simultaneous measurement of FHR and uterine activity came to be called electronic fetal monitoring or cardiotocography (CTG). Clinicians published papers describing the FHR wave-forms (patterns) formed on oscilloscopes or recorded on monitor paper, and relating the waveforms to fetal physiological responses. Investigators throughout the world made similar observations of FHR characteristics but developed different terms and definitions for the characteristics. International consensus conferences were held in an effort to standardize terminology, without success. Some agreement was achieved on deceleration pattern definitions but not on baseline variability or paper recording scales. Commercial monitors produced in the late 1960s increased the availability of the technology, and what was originally intended for use with high-risk laboring women was applied to low-risk laboring women and antepartum women. The use of EFM was encouraged after publications by Hon and later by Ralph Benson and colleagues, who had criticized the reliability and validity of FHR auscultation. Adjunct fetal assessment methods were also designed, including fetal scalp blood sampling in 1961, ultrasound of the fetal heart in 1964, the oxytocin challenge test (OCT) in 1975, the nonstress test (NST) in 1976, acoustical stimulation in 1977, scalp stimulation in 1982, biophysical profiles in 1985, and fetal pulse oximetry in 2000 (AWHONN, 2003).

Sandelowski (2000a,b) reported a detailed history of how performing EFM became part of the nurse's role and how nurses worked to integrate monitoring into childbirth and nursing care. Initially, nurses learned about EFM on site or at commercially sponsored training workshops. Educational publications on EFM for nurses began to appear in the 1960s. The FHR assessment that began as simply identifying the presence of an auditory heart signal has expanded to include assessing a continuous visual waveform of the changing FHR, recorded on paper or in some cases on a computer screen. Contemporary FHR assessment requires both auditory and visual skills.

The Present and the Future

Today's clinicians have access to peer-reviewed professional guidelines that outline standards for assessment, interpretation, and interventions, and to many excellent educational resources on fetal monitoring. However, providers and consumers continue to consider the advantages and limitations of widespread use of EFM. Consumers often read general news publications about the incidence of false alarms and subsequent cesarean sections with EFM (Cronin, 1996). The predominant "technological imperative" is thought to be causing an overly technocratic approach to birth (Davis-Floyd, Dumit, 1998). Clinicians repeatedly conclude that more research is needed on EFM reliability (observer agreement), validity (association with neonatal outcomes), and efficacy (preventive interventions that work). Randomized clinical trials have shown that neonatal outcomes are equivalent with either EFM or intermittent auscultation assessment in labors of low-risk women; thus auscultation skills are now frequently taught along with EFM skills. However, in most research trials, the nurse-to-fetus ratio reported for intermittent auscultation was 1:1 (Feinstein et al, 2000). This evidence-based ratio may not be possible with current nursing shortages and cost containment.

Contemporary computer technologies include networked central surveillance of EFM, electronic display and storage of the FHR tracing, integration of fetal physiological measurements (heart rate, oxygen saturation, fetal movement) and maternal physiological measurements (heart rate, oxygen saturation, blood pressure), wireless transmission of tracings, and fully electronic documentation in clinical information systems. Wireless technologies support FHR monitoring with maternal ambulation and use of water-filled tubs in labor. Health care systems are moving toward paperless environments, including a paperless FHR tracing. Computer algorithms can objectively identify tracing characteristics according to preprogrammed tracing definitions, sound alerts for identified characteristics, and even prompt tracing interpretation. This objectivity of automated computer analysis has improved research on FHR characteristics and practice interventions.

In the future, providers will need collaborative strategies for integrating increasingly complex biotechnologies and information technologies into best practices. The involvement of clinicians will be essential in researching the strengths and limitations of human and computer capabilities. When using technology such as EFM, clinicians will need to support interdisciplinary standardization, education, and competence validation.

References

American College of Obstetricians and Gynecologists (ACOG), American Academy of Pediatrics (AAP): *Neonatal encephalopathy and cerebral palsy: Defining the pathogenesis and pathophysiology,* Washington, DC, 2003, The College and the Academy.

Association of Women's Health, Obstetric and Neonatal Nurses (AWHONN): *Fetal heart monitoring principles and practices,* ed 3, Dubuque, Iowa, 2003, Kendall/Hunt.

Badawi N, Kurinczuk J, Keogh JM, et al: Intrapartum risk factors for new-born encephalopathy: The Western Australian case-control study, *BMJ* 317(7172):1554-1558, 1998.

Centers for Disease Control and Prevention (CDC): Births: Final data for 2000, *Natl Vital Stat Rep* 50(5):1-101, 2002.

Cronin B: Health report: The bad news, *Time,* 35, March 18, 1996.

Davis-Floyd R, Dumit J: *Cyborg babies,* New York, 1998, Routledge.

Feinstein N, Sprague A, Trepanier M: *Fetal heart rate auscultation,* Washington, DC, 2000, Association of Women's Health, Obstetric, and Neonatal Nurses.

Freeman RK, Garite TJ, Nageotte MP: *Fetal heart rate monitoring,* Baltimore, 2003, Williams and Wilkins

Hankins GD, Speer M: Defining the pathogenesis and pathophysiology of neonatal encephalopathy and cerebral palsy, *Obstet Gynecol* 102(3): 628-636, 2003.

MacLennan A: A template for defining a causal relationship between acute intrapartum events and cerebral palsy: International consensus statement, *BMJ* 319(7216):1054-1059, 1999.

National Institute for Child Health and Human Development Research Planning Workshop (NICHD): Electronic fetal heart rate monitoring research guidelines for interpretation, *Am J Obstet Gynecol* 177(6): 1385-1390, 1997.

Sandelowski M: Retrofitting technology to nursing: The case of electronic fetal monitoring, *J Obstet Gynecol Neonatal Nurs* 29(3):316-324, 2000a.

Sandelowski M: *Devices and desires: Gender, technology and American nursing,* Chapel Hill, NC, 2000b, University of North Carolina Press.

Physiological Basis for Monitoring

2

Electronic fetal monitoring provides a tool for assessment of utero-fetoplacental physiological exchange and the adequacy of fetal oxygenation. Characteristic fetal heart rate patterns occur as the result of hypoxic and nonhypoxic stresses or stimulation to the uterofetoplacental unit. Therefore it is important to have a basic understanding of the factors involved in fetal oxygenation, including uterofetoplacental circulation and the physiology of fetal heart rate regulation.

Uterofetoplacental Circulation

The placenta serves as a liaison between the fetal and the maternal circulations. The chorionic villi are tiny vascular branches of the placenta that extend into the intervillous space. Maternal blood spurts upward from the uterine spiral arterioles and spreads laterally into the intervillous space, completely surrounding and bathing the villi. The exchange of gases and substances occurs through the capillaries at the tips of the villi within the intervillous space (Figure 2-1). The oxygenated and nutrient-rich fetal blood is subsequently delivered to the fetus through the umbilical vein. Oxygen-poor and waste product–rich blood returns to the placental chorionic villi through the two umbilical arteries (Figure 2-2). Although maternal and fetal blood are separated by a thin membrane and do not mix, several mechanisms occur whereby substances are exchanged across this placental membrane.

Mechanisms Occurring Within the Intervillous Space

At term, some 700 to 800 ml of blood (10% to 15% of maternal cardiac output) perfuses the uterus each minute. Approximately 80% of this is within the intervillous space. Several mechanisms occur within the intervillous space. It acts as a depot for the exchange of oxygen and nutrients and provides for the elimination of waste products. Together with the chorionic villi, it functions as a fetal lung, gastrointestinal tract, kidney, skin (for heat exchange), infection barrier, and moderator of acid–base balance. Substances are exchanged by diffusion, active transport, bulk flow, pinocytosis, and leakage (Parer, 1997). Descriptions of these mechanisms and the substances are listed in Table 2-1.

Exchange of Gases

Transport and transfer of respiratory gases are of critical importance to fetal survival. Oxygen and carbon dioxide exchange are

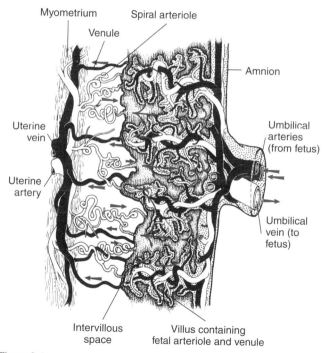

Figure 2-1

Schema of placenta. As maternal blood enters the intervillous space, it spurts from the uterine spiral arterioles and spreads laterally through the space. *White vessels* carry oxygenated blood. *Black vessels* carry oxygen-poor blood.

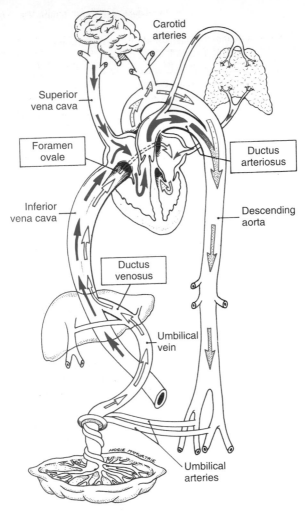

Figure 2-2

Fetal circulation. Oxygenated and nutrient-rich blood is carried to the fetus by the umbilical vein to the fetal heart. Oxygen-poor and waste product–rich blood circulates back to the placenta via the umbilical arteries. Three anatomic shunts (the ductus venosus, the foramen ovale, and the ductus arteriosus) permit fetal blood to bypass the liver and lungs.

(From Bloom RS: Delivery room resuscitation of the newborn. In Fanaroff AA, Martin RJ, editors: *Neonatal-perinatal medicine: Diseases of the fetus and infant,* ed 7, St Louis, 2002, Mosby.)

Table 2-1 Mechanisms occurring within the intervillous space

Mechanism	Description	Substances
Diffusion	Passage of substances from a region of higher concentration to one of lower concentration along a concentration gradient that is passive and requires no energy	Oxygen Carbon dioxide Small ions (sodium chloride) Lipids Fat-soluble vitamins Many drugs
Facilitated diffusion	Passage of substances on the basis of a concentration gradient; carrier molecule involved	Glucose Carbohydrates
Active transport	Passage of substances from one area to another against a concentration gradient; carrier molecules and energy are required	Amino acids Water-soluble vitamins Large ions (calcium, iron, iodine)
Bulk flow	Transfer of substances by a hydrostatic or osmotic gradient	Water Dissolved electrolytes
Pinocytosis	Transfer of minute, engulfed particles across a cell	Immune globulins Serum proteins
Breaks and leakage	Small breaks in the placental membrane allowing passage of substances	Maternal or fetal blood cells and plasma (potentially resulting in isoimmunization)

complex processes that depend on many physiological and biochemical factors. These include intervillous space blood flow, diffusing capacity of the placenta, placental area and vascularity, permeability of the placental membrane, diffusion distance, oxygen tension in uterine and umbilical blood vessels, hemoglobin affinity for oxygen, hemoglobin concentrations in maternal and fetal blood, and fetal umbilical cord blood flow. Alterations in an exchange mechanism may adversely affect the fetus by decreasing the transfer of oxygen to and carbon dioxide from the fetus.

A description of the factors affecting the exchange of gases follows. Intervillous space blood flow has already been described.

Diffusing capacity of placenta

The diffusing capacity of the placenta is its ability to transport oxygen from the placenta to the fetus. The rate of oxygen transport is dependent on the rate of blood flow and a concentration gradient. Oxygen diffuses from the maternal blood, which has a higher partial pressure, to the fetal blood, which has a lower partial pressure. The diffusing capacity is also affected by the surface area and thickness of the placental barrier: the larger the surface and the smaller the distance, the greater is the diffusing capacity (Meschia, 1999).

Maternal and fetal blood flow rates can be altered by a decrease in maternal blood pressure (as occurs with supine hypotension and following conduction anesthesia such as spinal, caudal, or epidural anesthesia), excessive maternal exercise, uterine polysystole or hypertonus, or decreased placental surface area (abruptio placentae or infarcts). The blood flow rate can also be altered by an increase in blood pressure, such as occurs with preeclampsia or vasoconstricting drugs (Parer, 1997).

Placental area

The larger and more vascular the placenta, the greater is the amount of each substance that can be transferred between woman and fetus. Reduced placental area is associated with abruptio placentae, maternal hypertension, maternal diabetes, maternal vascular disease, fetal growth restriction, intrauterine infection, placenta previa, placental infarctions, and circumvallate placenta.

Permeability of placental membrane

Membrane permeability is directly affected by characteristics of both the placental membrane and the substance that is diffusing. The physicochemical characteristics of a substance that determine its ability to pass through a membrane are its molecular weight, lipid solubility, degree of ionization (electrical charge), and protein-binding capability. These characteristics can enhance or limit the passage of potentially harmful drugs and other substances to the fetus (Blackburn, 2003).

Although the ability of a substance to cross the placenta cannot be accurately predicted by its molecular weight (MW), a rough approximation is that substances with an MW above 1000 *cannot* cross the placenta, whereas those with an MW below 1000 *can* (Parer, 1997). For example, heparin, with an MW of 6000, cannot cross the placenta, but warfarin (Coumadin), with an MW of 300, can cross and could anticoagulate the fetus. Lipid-soluble substances, such as lipoproteins, diazepam, and most sedatives, easily cross the placenta. Nonionized phenobarbital and the relatively un-ionized thiopental (MW of 264 and lipid soluble) easily cross the placenta (Blackburn, 2003; Parer, 1997). On the other hand, highly ionized (or electrically charged) particles are poorly diffusible; an example is succinylcholine, with an MW of only 361. Protein binding of a drug limits the amount that is available to transfer to the fetus. Ampicillin, which lacks significant binding to the protein albumin, easily crosses the placenta. However, carbon monoxide (firmly bound to maternal red blood cells) and dicloxacillin (firmly bound to plasma proteins) do not easily cross the placenta (Blackburn, 2003).

Substances that are highly permeable such as oxygen and carbon dioxide readily diffuse across the placental membrane. This process is dependent on the rate of blood flow: a decreased flow rate can reduce the exchange of gases.

Diffusion distance

An increased distance between the intervillous space and the fetal capillaries can decrease the transport of oxygen and exchange of gases. The diffusion distance is increased in several conditions as a result of villous hemorrhage, fibrin deposits, or villous edema, each of which serves to thicken the placental membrane. Fibrin deposits can occur with fetal dysmaturity (i.e., the fetus is small or large for gestational age), diabetes mellitus, and preeclampsia. Villous edema increases the diffusion distance in erythroblastosis fetalis and congenital syphilis. Villous hemorrhage and edema in maternal diabetes may also increase the diffusion distance (Freeman et al, 2003).

Oxygen tension

Oxygen tension (or partial pressure) in maternal arterial blood is determined by pulmonary function. Diminished function resulting from maternal disease processes or hypoventilation will decrease arterial oxygen tension (arterial Po_2, or Pao_2). Conditions that decrease arterial oxygen tension include chronic obstructive pulmonary diseases (asthma and emphysema), congestive heart failure, maternal congenital cardiac defects, and cystic fibrosis. The addition of inspired oxygen can increase arterial Po_2.

Oxygen transfer from maternal to fetal hemoglobin is regulated by the oxygen tension (or partial pressure) in the umbilical blood vessels. Generally, oxygen tension in the umbilical vessels is much lower than that in the maternal, or uterine, vessels. The median figures of maternal and fetal blood gas values are shown in Figure 2-3 (Helwig et al, 1996; Meschia, 1999; Parer, 1997).

The following factors compensate for the low fetal oxygen tension in the umbilical vessels (i.e., these factors ensure adequate oxygenation of the fetal tissues):

- Increased fetal cardiac output (three to four times that of the resting adult per kilogram of body weight) based on heart rate
- Increased oxygen-carrying capacity caused by high hemoglobin values (as compared with adult blood)
- Increased affinity of fetal blood for oxygen (as compared with adult blood), which results in a higher saturation of fetal hemoglobin at a given Po_2 based on the fetal hemoglobin dissociation curve
- The presence of anatomic fetal shunts: ductus venosus, foramen ovale, and ductus arteriosus

Hemoglobin and oxygen affinity

Hemoglobin concentrations in maternal and fetal blood differ at term. Maternal hemoglobin is approximately 12 g/dl, in contrast with fetal hemoglobin, which is about 15 g/dl. Each gram of hemoglobin is capable of combining with 1.34 ml of oxygen. This increased oxygen-carrying capacity of fetal blood and the high affinity of fetal blood for oxygen facilitate the transfer of oxygen from woman to fetus.

Oxygen saturation of hemoglobin is the relationship between the amount of oxygen that is carried on the hemoglobin and the amount of oxygen that *can* be carried. For example, a 98% saturation in the adult means that the hemoglobin is carrying 98% of its potential capacity. The amount of oxygen combined with hemoglobin depends on the partial pressure of oxygen dissolved in the arterial blood (Pao_2). The oxyhemoglobin saturations at different partial pressures vary, as demonstrated on a standard oxyhemoglobin dissociation curve (Figure 2-4). The curve is altered by changes in pH. This is known as the Bohr effect. The curve shifts to the right in the presence of an acidic pH and to the left in the presence of an alkaline pH. This changes the difference between the fetal and maternal curves and increases the gradient, which is beneficial for oxygen exchange.

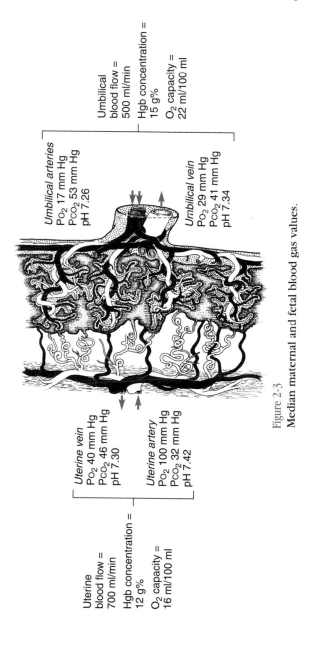

Figure 2-3
Median maternal and fetal blood gas values.

Umbilical
blood flow =
500 ml/min
Hgb concentration =
15 g%
O₂ capacity =
22 ml/100 ml

Umbilical arteries
Po₂ 17 mm Hg
Pco₂ 53 mm Hg
pH 7.26

Umbilical vein
Po₂ 29 mm Hg
Pco₂ 41 mm Hg
pH 7.34

Uterine vein
Po₂ 40 mm Hg
Pco₂ 46 mm Hg
pH 7.30

Uterine artery
Po₂ 100 mm Hg
Pco₂ 32 mm Hg
pH 7.42

Uterine
blood flow =
700 ml/min
Hgb concentration =
12 g%
O₂ capacity =
16 ml/100 ml

The oxygen saturation of hemoglobin can be measured in the woman by pulse oximetry (SpO_2). During the intrapartum period, fetal oxygen saturation ($FSpO_2$) can be measured by fetal pulse oximetry to better assess fetal status in the presence of a nonreassuring fetal heart rate (FHR) pattern as observed during electronic FHR monitoring. Fetal pulse oximetry monitoring is discussed in Chapter 6.

Umbilical blood flow

The mechanical force of a uterine contraction impedes intervillous space blood flow, exerts pressure directly on the fetus, and can

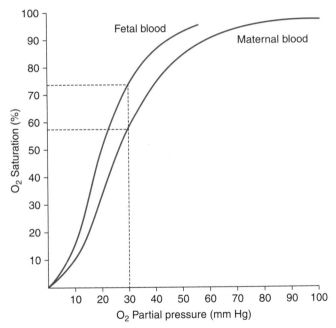

Figure 2-4
Oxygen dissociation curves of maternal and fetal blood. The vertical broken line illustrates the higher oxygen affinity of fetal blood. Fetal blood is more highly saturated with oxygen than is maternal blood at the same oxygen partial pressure.
(From Parer J: *Handbook of fetal heart rate monitoring,* Philadelphia, 1997, Saunders.)

occlude blood flow in both directions through the umbilical cord. Rapid fetal asphyxia with hypoxemia and acidosis can occur with entrapment and compression of the cord between fetal parts and the uterine wall. Transient cord compression occurs in about 40% of all labors, and the fetus is usually able to compensate in the intervals between contractions. However, during labor, if the cord prolapses or is short, knotted, or wrapped around fetal body parts, or if oligohydramnios is present, uncorrectable and prolonged variable deceleration of the FHR occurs. This is an obstetrical emergency, usually requiring immediate operative intervention, because fetal asphyxiation and death can occur. Amnioinfusion, the instillation of normal saline or lactated Ringer's solution through an intrauterine catheter (a discussion of which can be found in Chapter 6), can provide a buffer between fetal parts and the uterine wall and can relieve variable decelerations caused by cord compression. Variable decelerations are the characteristic FHR pattern associated with umbilical cord compression.

In summary, many factors determine the efficacy of fetal oxygenation through the exchange of gases. These include diffusing capacity of the placenta, placenta area, permeability of the placental membrane, diffusion distance, oxygen tension, hemoglobin affinity for oxygen, and umbilical blood flow. A summary of these factors and the maternal and fetal conditions that impede the exchange of gases are listed in Table 2-2.

Uterine Blood Flow

The passage of critical substances across the placenta is determined by uterine blood flow. The flow of blood increases as pregnancy progresses, so that by term about 700 ml of blood flows each minute. This volume is about 10% of the maternal cardiac output. About 85% of the total uterine blood flow circulates through the intervillous space and the remainder supplies the uterine musculature. Uterine blood flow is determined by uterine arterial and venous pressures and by uterine vascular resistance. Any impact on these three factors can alter uterine blood flow. For example, it is known that maternal rest in the lateral position increases uterine blood flow. Because no other practical means of improving uterine blood flow are known, it is important to understand and ameliorate, when possible, those factors that are known to decrease uterine blood flow. A discussion follows of some of the causes of decreased uterine blood flow, including maternal position,

Table 2-2 Factors affecting transport and transfer of maternal–fetal respiratory gases

Determinants of Fetal Oxygenation Processes	Conditions Impeding Exchange of Gases
Intervillous Space Blood Flow	
Rate and volume of blood flow directly affect the exchange of gases and nutrients	Maternal hypotension, hypertensive vascular disease, diabetes, regional anesthetics
Diffusing Capacity of Placenta	
Rate of oxygen transfer affected by the rate of blood flow and a concentration gradient (oxygen diffuses from maternal blood with a higher partial pressure to fetal blood with a lower partial pressure)	Maternal hypotension, exercise uterine hypertonus or polysystole, decreased placental surface area, maternal hypertension, preeclampsia
Area and Vascularity of Placenta	
The larger the surface area and the more vascular the placenta, the greater the amount of substances that can be transferred	Maternal smoking, preeclampsia, inadequate nutrition, diabetes with sclerotic changes, placenta previa, abruptio placentae, postmature fetus
Permeability of the Placental Membrane	
Membrane permeability is determined by molecular weight, lipid solubility, degree of ionization, and protein-binding capabilities of a substance	Decreased placental blood flow for any reason severely limits exchange of O_2 and CO_2, which are highly permeable substances
Diffusion Distance	
The transfer of oxygen may be decreased when there is a relatively large distance between the intervillous space and the fetal capillaries, as occurs with placenta edema, villous hemorrhage, and fibrin deposits	Maternal diabetes, preeclampsia, erythroblastosis fetalis, congenital syphilis, fetal dysmaturity

Table 2-2   Factors affecting transport and transfer of maternal–fetal respiratory gases—cont'd

Determinants of Fetal Oxygenation Processes	Conditions Impeding Exchange of Gases
Oxygen Saturation	
Relationship between amount of O_2 that is actually carried on the hemoglobin (Hgb) and the amount that can be carried varies at different partial pressures	Maternal hyperventilation, fetal hypoxemia, acid–base imbalance
Hemoglobin and Oxygen Affinity	
Fetal Hgb (15 g/dl) is higher than maternal Hgb (12 g/dl), which increases the oxygen-carrying capacity of fetal blood. The higher affinity of fetal blood for O_2 facilitates the transfer of O_2 to the fetus.	Maternal anemia due to hemoglobinopathies or hemorrhage (reduces available Hgb); fetal RhD alloimmunization
Maternal Arterial Oxygen Tension	
Maternal pulmonary function determines oxygen tension in maternal arterial blood. O_2 transfer from maternal to fetal Hgb is regulated by lower arterial Po_2 in umbilical vessels than in maternal blood vessels. Other compensating factors for low fetal Po_2 are increased fetal cardiac output based on FHR, increased O_2-carrying capacity, higher saturation of fetal Hgb, and anatomic shunts.	Maternal pulmonary dysfunction or pathology: chronic obstructive pulmonary disease, congestive heart failure, cystic fibrosis, chronic asthma, hypoventilation (particularly due to breath-holding)
Umbilical Blood Flow	
Determines adequacy of transport of blood between fetus and uteroplacental unit	Uterine hypertonus, uterine tachysystole, entrapment or compression of umbilical cord

Continued

Table 2-2   Factors affecting transport and transfer of maternal–fetal respiratory gases—cont'd

Determinants of Fetal Oxygenation Processes	Conditions Impeding Exchange of Gases
Uterine Blood Flow	
Affects passage of critical substances across placenta. Rate of flow is determined by uterine arterial and venous pressures and by uterine vascular resistance	Maternal position (causing supine hypotensive syndrome), excessive maternal exercise, uterine contractions or hypertonus, decreased surface area of placenta, conduction anesthesia (resulting in maternal hypotension), and maternal hypertension

exercise, uterine contractions, uterine hypertonus, surface area of placenta, conduction anesthesia, and hypertension.

Maternal position

A decrease in blood flow to the uterus can occur when the woman is in the dorsal recumbent position. The gravid uterus lies on the woman's vertebral column, exerting pressure on the great vessels, particularly the inferior vena cava. This pressure can compress the vessel, decreasing the volume of blood returning to the heart and producing a decrease in maternal cardiac output, hypotension, and a decrease in uterine blood flow. This mechanism is called supine hypotensive syndrome.

Maternal exercise

Maternal exercise has significant benefits for the woman and fetus, including the improvement of maternal fitness, shorter labors, and fewer perinatal complications (Hale, Milne, 1996; Riemann, Kanstrup Hansen, 2000). Physiological responses include increased oxygen consumption, redistribution of blood flow from the viscera to the skin and skeletal muscles, reduction in utero-ovarian blood flow, altered venous pooling, and changes in cardiac output and stroke volume. Compensatory mechanisms, however, help to maintain oxygen availability to the fetus during maternal exercise (Blackburn, 2003). For example, uterine blood flow is decreased significantly more than placental blood flow; however, uterine oxygen uptake increases to maintain stable oxygen consumption (Hartman, Bung, 1999). Maternal hemotocrit rises during exercise, increasing the maternal oxygen-carrying capacity. Alterations in venous blood return that are attributed to the progressive enlargement of the fetus and the uterus may be demonstrated by maternal dizziness and orthostatic hypotension. In late pregnancy, fatigue and dyspnea are observed as exercise tolerance decreases.

The fetal heart rate usually increases by 5 to 25 beats per minute (bpm) following maternal exercise and returns to pre-exercise values within 15 minutes (after moderate exercise) and 30 minutes (after strenuous exercise) (Hale, Milne, 1996; Riemann, Kanstrup Hansen, 2000). Exercise should be discontinued and the primary healthcare provider notified when maternal heart and respiratory rates do not return to resting rates within 15 minutes after exercise or in the presence of bleeding, shortness of breath, faintness, or back or pubic pain (Blackburn, 2003). Other warning signs to terminate exercise while pregnant include chest pain, dizziness, headache, muscle weakness, calf pain, and regular uterine contractions (AAP, ACOG, 2002).

Uterine contractions

Uterine contractions cause a decrease in the rate of perfusion of maternal blood through the intervillous space. Angiographic studies demonstrating this have shown impaired filling of the lobules with contrast medium during uterine contractions. In addition, fetal arterial blood oxygen tension (Pao_2) decreases following the onset of each uterine contraction. The fetus, in most gestations, seems well able to compensate for these relatively minor stresses. However, in pregnancies with risk factors, when the margin of fetal reserve is low, uterine contractions can cause some degree of hypoxia and commensurate decreases in the FHR, known as late decelerations. Recognition and treatment of late decelerations are described in Chapter 5.

To avoid compounding these stresses, it is important that the uterus relax adequately between contractions, that contractions not be excessively long, and that the tonus not rise. Intrauterine pressure between contractions—resting tone (tonus)—ranges from 10 to 15 mm Hg. During contractions, intrauterine pressure ranges from 30 mm Hg to more than 80 mm Hg, with an intensity of 50 mm Hg to more than 100 mm Hg at the peak of the contraction. Angiographic studies show a cessation of maternal blood flow to the intervillous space with intrauterine pressures of 50 to 60 mm Hg during normal labor contractions.

It is thought that the fetus receives most of the oxygen and nutrients and eliminates most of the carbon dioxide (CO_2) between contractions while the uterus is at rest. Thus a healthy fetus with a normal placenta subjected to frequent contractions with inadequate uterine relaxation can become hypoxic and acidotic.

Uterine hypertonus

Uterine hypertonus—excessively high intrauterine pressure—can also cause the fetus to experience stress. Uterine hypertonus may occur spontaneously in some women, particularly in those with a much distended uterus as a result of multiple gestations, hydramnios, or macrosomia. However, hypertonus is most frequently caused by uterine hyperstimulation with oxytocin during induction or augmentation of labor. In some sensitive women, oxytocin produces hypertonus, characterized by high intrauterine pressure with absence of relaxation for a prolonged period. Overstimulation with oxytocin can also result in tetanic contractions, uterine tachysystole (excessive frequency of uterine contractions), and signs of fetal intolerance to labor.

Abruptio placentae causes the greatest degree of uterine hyperactivity, whether hypertonus, tachysystole, or sustained uterine contraction. The hyperactivity and loss of placental surface area contribute to the appearance of a nonreassuring tracing. In preeclampsia, uterine resting tone is elevated because of vasoconstriction, and there is usually an increase in the frequency and intensity of uterine contractions (Freeman et al, 2003). In addition, the following factors can decrease uterine blood flow, interfere with placental perfusion, and stress the fetus:

- Contractions lasting longer than 90 seconds
- Periods of relaxation between contractions that are less than 30 seconds
- Inadequate decrease in intrauterine pressure between contractions

Surface area of placenta

The potential for fetal hypoxia is increased with any reduction in the placental surface area. Abruptio placentae is a clear example of this. Reduced placental area exposes the fetus to uteroplacental insufficiency and is associated with infarcts (as in hypertensive or prolonged pregnancies), maternal vascular disease, maternal diabetes, intrauterine infection, placenta previa, or circumvallate placenta.

Conduction anesthesia

Maternal hypotension caused by sympathetic blockade occurring with conduction anesthesia reduces blood flow in the intervillous space. Restoration of uterine blood flow is usually achieved by positional changes and expansion of maternal blood volume. Prehydration for women who are about to receive conduction anesthesia should be considered. Ephedrine may also be required to restore maternal blood pressure (Freeman et al, 2003).

Hypertension

Whether maternal hypertension is essential or pregnancy induced, there is an increase in vascular resistance, resulting in a decrease in uterine blood flow.

In summary, the factors that are known to impede uterine blood flow include maternal supine position, supine hypotensive syndrome, excessive maternal exercise, uterine contractions, uterine hypertonus, decreased surface area of the placenta, conduction anesthesia, and hypertension. Appropriate interventions can improve uterine blood flow. Examples of such interventions are lateral maternal positioning, avoidance of excessive exercise, avoidance of uterine hyperstimulation with oxytocin, rehydration or use of volume expanders, and use of antihypertensive agents.

Physiology of Fetal Heart Rate Regulation

The average FHR at term is 140 beats per minute. The normal range is 110 to 160 bpm. Earlier in gestation, the FHR is slightly higher, with the average being approximately 160 bpm at 20 weeks' gestation (Freeman et al, 2003). The rate progressively decreases as the fetus reaches term.

Regulatory control of the FHR depends on multiple factors (Parer, 1997), as described in Table 2-3. The cerebral cortex, hypothalamus, and medulla oblongata are components of the central nervous system that influence the FHR. The autonomic nervous system has two major divisions: the parasympathetic and sympathetic nervous systems. The vagus nerve, which innervates

Table 2-3   Regulatory control of fetal heart rate (FHR)

Factors Regulating FHR	Location
Parasympathetic division of autonomic nerve system	Vagus (10th cranial) nerve fibers supply sinoatrial (SA) and atrioventricular (AV) nodes
Sympathetic division of autonomic nervous system	Nerves widely distributed in myocardium
Baroceptors	Stretch receptors in aortic arch and carotid sinus at the junction of the internal and external carotid arteries
Chemoceptors	Peripheral—in carotid and aortic bodies
	Central—in medulla oblongata
Central nervous system	Cerebral cortex
	Hypothalamus
	Medulla oblongata
Hormonal regulation	Adrenal medulla (catecholamines)

Action	Effect
Stimulation causes release of acetylcholine at myoneural synapse	Decreases FHR Maintains short-term variability
Stimulation causes release of norepinephrine at synapse	Increases FHR Increases strength of myocardial contraction Increases cardiac output
Responds to increase in blood pressure by stimulating stretch receptors to send impulses via vagus or glossopharyngeal nerve to midbrain, producing vagal response and slowing heart activity	Decreases FHR Decreases blood pressure Decreases cardiac output
Responds to a marked peripheral decrease in O_2 and increase in CO_2	Produces bradycardia, sometimes with increased variability
Central chemoceptors respond to decreases in O_2 tension and increases in CO_2 tension in blood and/or cerebrospinal fluid	Produces tachycardia and increase in blood pressure with decrease in variability
Responds to fetal movement	Increases reactivity and variability
Responds to fetal sleep	Decreases reactivity and variability
Regulates and coordinates autonomic activites (sympathetic and parasympathetic)	
Mediates cardiac and vasomotor reflex center by controlling heart action and blood vessel diameter	Maintains balance between cardioacceleration and cardiodeceleration: modulates variability
Releases epinephrine and norepinephrine with severe fetal hypoxia producing sympathetic response	Increases FHR Increases strength of myocardial contraction and blood pressure Increases cardiac output

Continued

Table 2-3   Regulatory control of fetal heart rate (FHR)—cont'd

Factors Regulating FHR	Location
Hormonal regulation—cont'd	Adrenal cortex
	Pituitary neurohypophysis (vasopressin)
	Renal juxtaglomerular cells (renin-agniotensin II)
Blood volume/capillary fluid shift	Fluid shift between capillaries and interstitial spaces
Intraplacental pressures	Intervillous space
Frank-Starling mechanism	Based on stretching of myocardium by increased inflow of venous blood into right atrium

Action	Effect
Low fetal blood pressure stimulates release of aldosterone, decreases sodium output, increases water retention, which increases circulating blood volume	Maintains homeostasis of blood volume
Produces vasoconstriction of nonvital vascular beds in the asphyxiated fetus to increase blood pressure	Distributes blood flow to maintain FHR and variability; linked to sinusoidal pattern
Released when intra-arterial volume low	Stimulates vasoconstriction to maintain blood pressure
Responds to elevated blood pressure by causing fluid to move out of capillaries and into interstitial spaces	Decreases blood volume and blood pressure
Responds to low blood pressure by causing fluid to move out of interstitial space into capillaries	Increases blood volume and blood pressure
Fluid shift between fetal and maternal blood is based on osmotic and blood pressure gradients; maternal blood pressure is about 100 mm Hg and fetal blood pressure about 55 mm Hg; therefore balance is probably maintained by some compensatory factor	Regulates blood volume and blood pressure
In the adult the myocardium is stretched by an increased inflow of blood, causing the heart to contract with greater force than before and pump out more blood; the adult then is able to increase cardiac output by increasing heart rate and stroke volume; this mechanism is not well developed in the fetus	Cardiac output is dependent on heart rate in the fetus: $\downarrow$ FHR = $\downarrow$ cardiac output $\uparrow$ FHR = $\uparrow$ cardiac output

the sinoatrial (SA) node and the atrioventricular (AV) node of the fetal heart, is the primary component of the parasympathetic nervous system. Stimulation of the vagus nerve produces cardio-deceleration. Stimulation of the sympathetic nervous system results in cardioacceleration.

Baroreceptors are stretch receptors or pressoreceptors in the aortic arch and carotid sinus that respond to changes in blood pressure, effecting a change in the FHR. Peripheral chemore-ceptors located in carotid and aortic bodies can effect bradycardia, and central chemoreceptors located in the medulla oblongata can effect tachycardia. A schema of the relationship of these factors in regulating FHR is depicted in Figure 2-5. Other factors that may

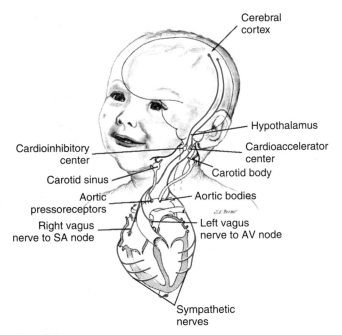

Figure 2-5
Relationships of the factors that control the fetal heart rate: the central nervous system (cerebral cortex, hypothalamus, medulla oblongata), the parasympathetic (cardioinhibitory center) and sympathetic divisions (cardioacceleratory center) of the autonomic nervous system, baroreceptors, and chemoreceptors.

influence the FHR are disturbances such as hyperthermia (resulting in tachycardia) and hypothermia (resulting in bradycardia).

Fetal Heart Rate Response

The fetal heart rate responds to alterations in uteroplacental circulation, umbilical blood flow, fetal circulation, and respiratory gas exchange. The most common interruption of oxygen delivery to the fetus is an acute decrease in uterine or umbilical blood flow. Under normal conditions, the fetus compensates for short-term transient decreases in Po_2 without altering normal metabolic function (King, Parer, 2000). The terms *placental* and *fetal reserve* describe the oxygen reserve that allows the fetus to compensate for these transient changes. As the available oxygen decreases below a critical threshold, the fetus develops anaerobic metabolism. This results in the production of lactic acid, which transfers across the placenta and eventually causes acidemia and metabolic acidosis (Parer, 1997). Late decelerations when accompanied by minimal variability are the characteristic fetal heart rate pattern associated with metabolic acidosis.

Compression of the umbilical cord is usually a temporary phenomenon during the course of labor, but, when repetitive with a decrease in variability and a rise in baseline rate, it can result in respiratory acidosis. Variable decelerations are the characteristic fetal heart rate pattern associated with cord compression and are discussed in Chapter 5.

Risk Factors

Multiple antepartum and intrapartum maternal and fetal factors can increase maternal and fetal/neonatal risk. The majority of these factors are associated with uteroplacental insufficiency. Early identification is needed to provide direction for patient care management. Identification of specific risk factors should prompt the health care provider to perform a focused assessment and judicious monitoring of the woman to avoid an undesirable or adverse outcome.

These factors are grouped into three major categories: medical history and conditions, obstetrical history and conditions, and intrapartum factors. This list in Box 2-1 provides the common factors that place the woman and fetus/newborn at risk, but it is not exhaustive.

Box 2-1   Maternal and Fetal Risk Factors

These factors are categorized into three major categories: medical history and conditions, obstetrical history and conditions, and intrapartum factors. This list provides the more common factors that place the woman and fetus/newborn at risk. Identification of risk factors is important to plan for patient care management.

Medical History and Conditions

- Anemia
- Antiphospholipid syndrome
- Asthma
- Cancer
- Cardiac disease
- Collagen diseases (e.g., systemic lupus erythematosus [SLE], rheumatoid arthritis, scleroderma)
- Condylomata, extensive
- Diabetes mellitus, type 1 or 2
- Domestic violence/intimate partner abuse
- Drug addiction or alcohol abuse
- Epilepsy
- Family history of genetic disorders
- Hemoglobinopathy
- Human immunodeficiency virus (HIV)
- Hypertension
- Immunological disorders (autoimmune and alloimmune)
- Neurological disorder
- Nutritional status, poor
- Psychiatric illness
- Pulmonary disorders
- Renal disease
- Scoliosis
- Smoking
- Thromboembolic disease
- Thyroid disease
- Urinary tract infection
- Uterine leiomyomata or malformation

Obstetrical History and Conditions

- Abnormal fetal presentation
- Age >35 at delivery
- Decreased fetal movement
- Emotional instability
- Fetal anomalies (e.g., anencephaly)
- Fetal cardiac malformation
- Fetal growth restriction
- Gestational age >41 weeks
- Gestational diabetes
- HELLP (hemolysis, elevated liver enzymes, and low platelet counts) syndrome

Box 2-1   Maternal and Fetal Risk Factors—cont'd

- Herpes, active lesions
- Hydramnios
- Incompetent cervix
- Intrauterine growth restriction
- Isoimmunization
- Lack of prenatal care
- Low income
- Marginal separation of placenta
- Multiparity
- Multiple gestation, especially with discordant growth
- Nonimmune hydrops
- Oligohydramnios
- Preeclampsia
- Pregnancy-related hypertension
- Premature rupture of membranes
- Preterm labor
- Previous cesarean delivery
- Prior fetal structural or genetic disorder
- Prior low birth weight (<2500 g)
- Prior neonatal death
- Prior preterm delivery
- Prior unexplained fetal death
- Proteinuria
- Sexually transmitted disease (STD), untreated
- Systemic disease that has an adverse impact on pregnancy

- Vaginal bleeding

Intrapartum Factors
- Abnormal antenatal test
- Abruptio placentae
- Assisted vaginal delivery, vacuum or forceps
- Amnionitis
- Dysfunctional labor pattern
- General anesthesia
- Hemorrhage
- Illicit drug use
- Low birth weight, expected or actual
- Maternal fever
- Meconium in amniotic fluid
- Nonreassuring fetal heart rate pattern
- Oxytocin augmentation or induction of labor
- Placenta previa
- Postterm fetus
- Precipitous labor
- Preterm fetus
- Prolapsed umbilical cord
- Prolonged rupture of membranes >24 hours
- Prolonged second stage of labor
- Shoulder dystocia
- Uterine hyperactivity/ tetany
- Uterine rupture

In summary, determining factors in the fetal response to labor include regulatory control of the FHR, the quality and efficacy of uteroplacental circulation, umbilical blood flow, respiratory gas exchange, and fetal circulation. An understanding of these factors forms the basis for fetal heart rate and uterine activity monitoring.

References

American Academy of Pediatrics (AAP), American College of Obstetricians and Gynecologists (ACOG): *Guidelines for perinatal care,* Washington, DC, 2002, The Academy and the College.

Blackburn ST: *Maternal, fetal, and neonatal physiology: A clinical perspective,* ed 2, St Louis, 2003, Mosby.

Bloom RS: Delivery room resuscitation of the newborn. In Fanaroff AA, Martin RJ, editors: *Neonatal-perinatal medicine: Diseases of the fetus and infant,* ed 7, St Louis, 2002, Mosby.

Freeman RK, Garite TJ, Nageotte MP: *Fetal heart rate monitoring,* ed 3, Baltimore, 2003, Williams & Wilkins.

Hale RW, Milne L: The elite athlete and exercise in pregnancy, *Semin Perinatal* 20(4):277-281, 1996.

Hankins GD, Speer M: Defining the pathogenesis and pathophysiology of neonatal encephalopathy and cerebral palsy, *Obstet Gynecol* 102(3): 628-636, 2003.

Hartmann S, Bung P: Physical exercise during pregnancy: Physiological considerations and recommendations, *J Perinat Med* 27(3):204-215, 1999.

Helwig IT, Parer JT, Kilpatrick SJ, et al: Umbilical cord blood acid–base state: What is normal? *Am J Obstet Gynecol* 174(6):1807-1812, 1996.

King T, Parer JT: The physiology of fetal heart rate patterns and perinatal asphyxia, *J Perinat Neonatal Nurs* 14(3):19-39, 2000.

Meschia G: Placental respiratory gas exchange and fetal oxygenation. In Creasy RK, Resnik R, editors: *Maternal–fetal medicine,* ed 4, Philadelphia, 1999, Saunders.

Parer J: *Handbook of fetal heart rate monitoring,* Philadelphia, 1997, Saunders.

Riemann MK, Kanstrup Hansen IL: Effects on the foetus of exercise in pregnancy, *Scand J Med Sci Sports* 10(1):12-19, 2000.

Instrumentation for Fetal Heart Rate and Uterine Activity Monitoring

3

The goal of fetal heart rate (FHR) monitoring is to detect signs that warn of potential adverse events so as to provide intervention in a timely manner. The FHR can be monitored by intermittent auscultation or by electronic means with an external or internal device. This chapter describes the devices that can be used to monitor the FHR and includes information on uterine activity monitoring, central display terminals, and telemetry. In addition, factors to be considered before purchasing an electronic monitor are provided.

Auscultation of Fetal Heart Rate

Description

A technique that can be used in addition to electronic fetal monitoring (EFM) is auscultation of the FHR with a stethoscope, DeLee-Hillis fetoscope, Pinard stethoscope, and Doppler ultrasound device (Figure 3-1). Auscultation, a learned skill that improves with practice, is *not* electronic fetal monitoring without a tracing. It is a *counting* technique in which an instrument (or a listening device) is used to count the number of fetal heart beats occurring in a prescribed amount of time and evaluated at prescribed intervals of time. The rate obtained is utilized, along with other assessment data, to guide management and care of the maternal–fetal dyad.

If a *stethoscope* is used, the end should be turned so that the domed side of the stethoscope, rather than the flat side, is open to the connective tubing leading to the earpieces. The domed side is

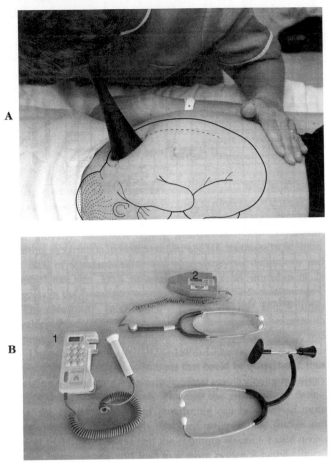

Figure 3-1
A, Auscultation of FHR with a Pinard stethoscope. Vertex left occipitoanterior. **B,** *1,* Ultrasound fetoscope; *2,* ultrasound stethoscope; *3,* DeLee-Hillis fetoscope.
(**A,** From Fraser DM, Cooper MA, editors: *Myles textbook for midwives,* ed 14, London, 2003, Churchill Livingstone. **B,** Courtesy Michael S. Clement, MD, Mesa, Ariz.)

then placed on the maternal abdomen over the area of maximum intensity. The *fetoscope* should be applied to the listener's head, because bone conduction amplifies the fetal heart sounds for counting. It is the ventricular fetal heart sounds that can be counted with the stethoscope and fetoscope. The *Doppler ultrasound* device transmits ultra-high-frequency sound waves to the moving interface of the fetal heart valves and deflects these back to the device, converting them into an electronic signal that can be counted. Auscultation is useful to establish the fetal heart rate before initiating electronic fetal monitoring, and to validate the electronic fetal heart rate.

Procedure	Rationale
1. Explain procedure to woman and support person.	1. Provides teaching opportunity and decreases anxiety
2. Perform Leopold's maneuvers (Figure 3-2) by palpating the maternal abdomen.	2. To identify fetal presentation and position
3. Apply ultrasound gel to device if using a Doppler ultrasound. Place the listening device over the area of maximum intensity (usually over the back of the fetus). If using the fetoscope, firm pressure may be needed.	3. To obtain the clearest and loudest sound (easier to count)
4. Count the maternal radial pulse.	4. To differentiate it from the fetal rate
5. Palpate the abdomen for the presence or absence of uterine activity.	5. To be able to count FHR between contractions
6. Count the FHR for 30 or 60 seconds between contractions.	6. To identify the baseline rate (best assessed in the absence of uterine activity)
7. Auscultate the FHR during a contraction, if possible, and for 30 seconds after the end of the contraction.	7. To identify the FHR during the contraction, as a response to the contraction and to assess for the absence or presence of increases or decreases in FHR

Continued on p. 38

Leopold's Maneuvers

Perform hand hygiene.

Explain procedure to woman.

Ask woman to empty bladder.

Position woman supine with one pillow under her head and with her knees slightly flexed.

Place small rolled towel under her right hip to displace uterus to left of major blood vessels (prevents supine hypotensive syndrome).

If right-handed, stand on woman's right, facing her:

1. Identify fetal part that occupies the fundus. The head feels round, firm, freely movable, and palpable by ballottement; the breech feels less regular and softer (identifies fetal lie [longitudinal or transverse] and presentation [cephalic or breech]; see figure below).

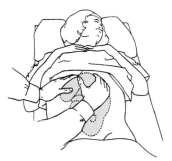

2. Using palmar surface of one hand, locate and palpate the smooth convex contour of the fetal back and the irregularities that identify the small parts (feet, hands, elbows). This assists in identifying fetal presentation (see figure below).

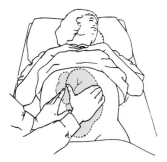

3. With the right hand, determine which fetal part is presenting over the inlet to the true pelvis. Gently grasp the lower pole of the uterus between the thumb and fingers, pressing in slightly (see figure below). If the head is presenting and not engaged, determine the attitude of the head (flexed or extended).

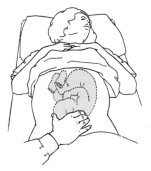

4. Turn to face the woman's feet. Using both hands, outline the fetal head (see figure below) with palmar surface of fingertips.

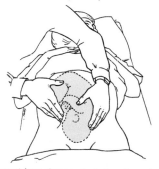

When presenting part has descended deeply, only a small portion of it may be outlined.

Palpation of cephalic prominence assists in identifying attitude of head. If the cephalic prominence is found on the same side as the small parts, the head must be flexed, and the vertex is presenting. If the cephalic prominence is on the same side as the back, the presenting head is extended and the face is presenting.

Determination of Point of Maximal Intensity of the Fetal Heart Rate

Perform hand hygiene.
Explain procedure to woman.

Continued

Perform Leopold's maneuvers.

Auscultate FHR on basis of fetal presentation. The PMI is the location where the FHR is heard the loudest, usually over the fetal back.

Chart fetal presentation, position, and lie; determine whether presenting part is flexed or extended, engaged or free floating. Use hospital's protocol for charting (e.g., "Vtx, LOA, floating").

Chart PMI of FHR using a two-line figure to indicate the four quadrants of the maternal abdomen, right upper quadrant (RUQ), left upper quadrant (LUQ), left lower quadrant (LLQ), and right lower quadrant (RLQ):

RUQ	LUQ
RLQ	LLQ

The umbilicus is the reference point for the quadrants (the point where the lines cross). The PMI for the fetus in vertex presentation, in general flexion with the back on the mother's right side, is commonly found in the mother's right lower quadrant and is recorded with an "X" or with the FHR as follows:

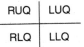

Figure 3-2
Leopold's maneuvers and determination of the points of maximum intensity (PMI) of the fetal heart rate.
(From Lowdermilk DL, Perry SE: *Maternity & women's health care,* ed 8, St Louis, 2004, Mosby.)

Procedure—cont'd	Rationale—cont'd
8. When there are distinct discrepancies in FHR during listening periods, auscultate for a longer period during, after, and between contractions.	8. To identify changes from the baseline that indicate the need for another mode of FHR monitoring

Frequency of Auscultation

Regardless of the method used to assess FHR, the standard practice is to evaluate and record the heart rate at specific intervals.

There are currently no recommendations for FHR assessment in the *latent phase of labor* from the American College of Obstetricians and Gynecologists (ACOG), the Society of Obstetricians and Gynecologists of Canada (SOGC), or the Association of Women's Health, Obstetric and Neonatal Nurses (AWHONN). It is suggested by AWHONN that the FHR be assessed at least as often as maternal vital signs and more frequently if there is any change in condition.

The Royal College of Obstetricians and Gynecologists (RCOG, 2001) in England recommends intermittent auscultation at least every 15 minutes in the active stage of labor for a minimum of 60 seconds after a contraction, and every 5 minutes in the second stage of labor.

In the following chart, the frequency of auscultation and documentation of the fetal heart rate is based on AAP/ACOG guidelines (2002), SOGC standards (2002), and AWHONN (2003).

Stage of Labor	Low Risk	High Risk
Active phase	q 30 minutes	q 15 minutes
Second stage	q 15 minutes	q 5 minutes

On the basis of reviews of well-controlled studies, no differences in perinatal outcomes have been identified between intermittent auscultation and continuous electronic FHR monitoring (Vintzileos et al, 1995). This has been observed even in the presence of risk factors seen on admission or those appearing during the course of labor, when the FHR has been evaluated at the intervals described in the preceding chart (AAP, ACOG, 2002). It is important to note that the studies did employ *a ratio of one nurse to one patient,* which should be done if auscultation is used as the primary technique of FHR surveillance.

Auscultation of the FHR should occur *before* the following events occur:

- Administration of medications (including oxytocics and analgesics) or anesthetics
- Periods of ambulation
- Artificial rupture of membranes

The FHR should be assessed *immediately after* the following events occur:

- Rupture of membranes
- A change in the strength of the uterine contractions (resting tone increase, sustained contraction, or tachysystole)

- Vaginal examination
- A change in the dosage of oxytocics, and when a response to oxytocics is noted
- Administration of medications (during peak action period)
- Urinary catheterization
- Periods of ambulation
- A change in the dosage of analgesics and anesthetic agents, and when a response is noted

Many countries prefer intermittent auscultation to continuous electronic fetal monitoring in women without risk factors, as this promotes their mobility, is less distracting, and provides a more natural birthing experience without the use of electronic devices. Reliance on the electronic monitor is more prevalent in the United States, most likely because of staffing patterns, staffing mix, and the increased use of defensive practices in a litigious environment.

Documentation

Documentation of the FHR must be accompanied by other routine parameters that are assessed during labor, including uterine activity, maternal observations and assessment, and both maternal and fetal responses to interventions. It should be noted how long the heart rate was auscultated and whether this was before, during, and/or immediately after a uterine contraction. The rate, rhythm, and abrupt or gradual increases or decreases of the FHR during any part of this auscultated period should be described in relationship to uterine activity.

NOTE: It is *not* appropriate to describe auscultated FHR using the descriptive terms associated with electronic fetal monitoring because the majority of the EFM terms are *visual descriptions* of the patterns produced on the monitor tracing (e.g., early, late, and variable decelerations or variability). However, terms that are numerically defined, such as bradycardia and tachycardia, can be used.

Interpretation of Auscultated Fetal Heart Rate
Reassuring fetal heart rate

- FHR with a normal baseline range of 110 to 160 beats per minute (bpm)
- Regular rhythm (obtained between contractions), without wide fluctuations from the average rate
- Presence of increases from the baseline rate
- Absence of decreases from the baseline rate, assessed over a 10-minute period

Nonreassuring fetal heart rate

- A baseline FHR of <110 bpm or >160 bpm
- A decrease in the FHR from baseline, either during or after contractions
- Irregular rhythm
- Decreased FHR from baseline, during and within 30 seconds after contractions
- Abrupt or gradual decrease in baseline FHR

Management options of a nonreassuring fetal heart rate

- Increase frequency of auscultation
- Apply electronic fetal monitor to visualize pattern suspected or to assess baseline variability
- Intervene appropriately to promote uterine and umbilical blood flow, improve fetal oxygenation, and decrease uterine activity if excessive (AWHONN, 2003)
- Vibroacoustic stimulation with electronic monitoring to assess fetal response
- Notify health care provider as appropriate

If a nonreassuring fetal heart rate persists after attempts to correct it, or if ancillary tests are not appropriate, then an expeditious delivery may be considered by the health care provider.

Benefits and Limitations of Auscultation
Benefits

- Widely available and easy to use
- Less invasive
- Outcomes comparable to EFM with 1:1 nursing care
- Inexpensive
- Comfortable for the woman
- Provides freedom of movement for the woman
- Increases hands-on contact with the woman
- Allows FHR assessment during use of hydrotherapy

Limitations

- May be difficult to obtain FHR in some situations, such as polyhydramnios and maternal obesity
- Does not provide a permanent, documented record
- The counting of FHR is intermittent

- Cannot assess visual patterns of FHR variability or periodic changes
- Nonreassuring events may occur during unauscultated periods
- May not allow early detection of a nonreassuring fetal heart rate

In summary, auscultatory FHR monitoring has been found to be effective if performed in a consistent manner by a nurse caring for a woman according to the prescribed frequency. Because of the time- and labor-intensive nature of this method of monitoring, it may not always be an option in a busy unit that has the capability of continuous electronic FHR monitoring.

Electronic Fetal Monitoring
Overview

There are two modes of electronic monitoring. The external, or indirect, mode employs the use of external transducers placed on the maternal abdomen to assess FHR and uterine activity. The internal, or direct, mode uses a spiral electrode (to assess the FHR and variability) and an intrauterine pressure catheter (to assess uterine activity and intrauterine pressure) (Figures 3-3 to 3-5). In some countries, the electronic fetal monitor is called a cardiotocograph (CTG). The following chart compares the external and internal modes of monitoring and gives a brief description of the equipment used for each.

External Mode (Indirect)	Internal Mode (Direct)
Fetal heart rate	
Ultrasound (Doppler) transducer: High-frequency sound waves reflect mechanical action of fetal heart. This is the easiest and most reliable external method to use during the antepartum and intrapartum periods.	**Spiral electrode:** Electrode converts fetal electrocardiogram (ECG) (as obtained from presenting part) to FHR via cardiotachometer by measuring consecutive fetal R-wave intervals. This method can be used only when the membranes are ruptured and the cervix is sufficiently dilated during the intrapartum period. The electrode penetrates the fetal presenting part 1.5 mm, and it must be securely attached to ensure a good signal.

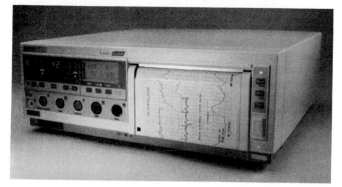

Figure 3-3
The Viridia 50 XM fetal/maternal monitor provides
measurement of fetal heart rate (FHR), uterine activity (UA),
gross fetal body movement, twin offset (to separate FHR
tracings of twins for easier interpretation), and maternal
parameters, including ECG, heart rate, noninvasive blood
pressure, and pulse oximetry. The Viridia 50 XMO monitors
the foregoing with the addition of fetal pulse oximetry.
(Courtesy Philips Medical Systems, Böblingen, Germany.)

Uterine activity

Tocotransducer: This instrument monitors the approximate frequency and duration of contractions by means of a pressure-sensing device applied to the abdomen. It can be used during antepartum and intrapartum periods.

Intrauterine catheter: This instrument monitors frequency, duration, and intensity of contractions, and resting tone. The catheter is compressed during contractions, placing pressure on a transducer tip or the strain gauge mechanism of a fluid-filled catheter and then converting the pressure into millimeters of mercury (mm Hg) on the uterine activity panel of the monitor tracing. It can be used only when the membranes are ruptured and the cervix is sufficiently dilated during intrapartum period. These catheters are available with a second lumen that can be used for amnioinfusion.

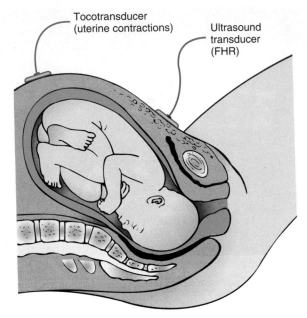

Figure 3-4
Placement of external transducers. The tocotransducer transmits uterine activity. The ultrasound transducer transmits fetal heart rate (FHR).
(From Lowdermilk DL, Perry SE: *Maternity & women's health care,* ed 8, St Louis, 2004, Mosby.)

Indications for Electronic Monitoring

Meta-analyses of clinical trials have not demonstrated improved infant morbidity or mortality with electronic fetal monitoring compared to intermittent auscultation of the fetal heart rate, even in high-risk pregnancies. Because of limitations in both budget and staff in the intrapartum setting, the ability to perform intermittent auscultation with a 1:1 nurse–patient ratio is severely restricted in the majority of health care facilities. Thus it is anticipated that intermittent or continuous electronic fetal monitoring will continue to be routinely used for specific indications as designated by the institution. These may include the following:

- Screening of women who present for admission
- On admission to the perinatal unit

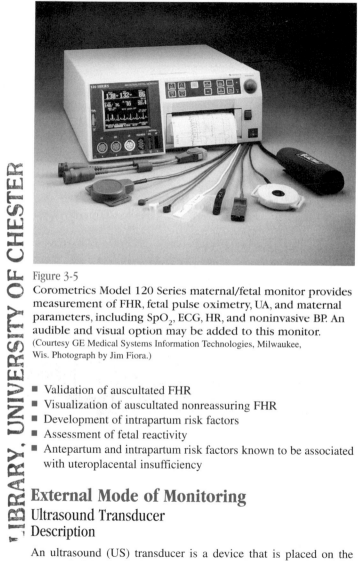

Figure 3-5
Corometrics Model 120 Series maternal/fetal monitor provides
measurement of FHR, fetal pulse oximetry, UA, and maternal
parameters, including SpO$_2$, ECG, HR, and noninvasive BP. An
audible and visual option may be added to this monitor.
(Courtesy GE Medical Systems Information Technologies, Milwaukee,
Wis. Photograph by Jim Fiora.)

- Validation of auscultated FHR
- Visualization of auscultated nonreassuring FHR
- Development of intrapartum risk factors
- Assessment of fetal reactivity
- Antepartum and intrapartum risk factors known to be associated
  with uteroplacental insufficiency

External Mode of Monitoring
Ultrasound Transducer
Description

An ultrasound (US) transducer is a device that is placed on the
maternal abdomen and transmits ultrasonic high-frequency sound
waves. As the ultrasound strikes a moving interface—in this case
the fetal heart—a signal is directed back to the transducer, activating

a tachometer. The rate of the moving interface, the fetal heart, is printed out on the upper part of the tracing or monitor strip, and a simultaneous indicator light or audible beep on the monitor is activated with each heartbeat. This Doppler signal can be affected by changes in the position of the transducer or the fetus. Changes in the direction of the sound beam during uterine contractions may cause a loss of signal and make the resulting tracing uninterpretable. Because ultrasound reflects the mechanical movement of the fetal heart, it cannot assess accurate short-term variability of the FHR. However, monitors with autocorrelation capability very closely approximate accurate short-term variability. Autocorrelation works by matching each incoming waveform with the previous one and repetitively analyzing small segments of those waveforms. Because autocorrelation enhances signal-to-noise levels, it may produce a false signal, showing an apparent heart rate in the absence of fetal cardiac motion (Freeman et al, 2003).

Some monitors have dual ultrasound channels for the simultaneous monitoring of twins and multiples. The two readings may be offset so that each twin's FHR can more easily be identified (see p. 65) (Figure 3-6).

The ultrasound transducer can be used to monitor FHR during both antepartum and intrapartum periods. Correct placement of the ultrasound transducer depends on maternal cooperation and operator skill, because the transducer must usually be repositioned

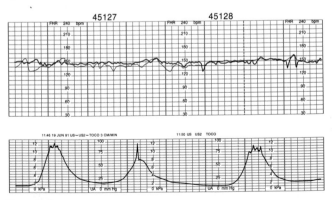

Figure 3-6
Dual ultrasound heart rate monitoring strip demonstrates the simultaneous external monitoring of twins.
(Courtesy GE Medical Systems Information Technologies, Milwaukee, Wis.)

when the maternal position changes. Artifacts and erratic tracings may result from a number of causes, such as increased variability, halving or doubling of the FHR by the monitor, recording of maternal heart rate, fetal arrhythmias, and fetal or maternal movement.

Placement of ultrasound transducer

The following chart provides a step-by-step approach for the use of the ultrasound transducer.

Procedure	Rationale
1. Explain the procedure to the woman and her family.	1. To allay anxiety
2. Gather necessary equipment: fetal monitor, ultrasound transducer, apparatus for either tocotransducer or intrauterine catheter (to assess uterine activity), ultrasonic coupling gel, and abdominal belt.	2. To ensure that all equipment is readily accessible
3. Position the woman in a comfortable semilateral position.	3. To maximize uteroplacental blood flow by avoiding supine hypotension syndrome
4. Perform Leopold's maneuvers (see Figure 3-2).	4. To determine fetal position, lie, and presentation
5. Align and insert the ultrasound transducer plug into the appropriate monitor port (labeled cardio, or US for ultrasound).	5. To provide connection without damaging connector pins (could result in a faulty signal)
6. Apply ultrasound gel to the underside of the transducer placed on the maternal abdomen.	6. To aid in the transmission of ultrasound waves
7. Place the transducer on the abdomen, preferably over the fetal back or below the level of the umbilicus for a full-term pregnancy of cephalic presentation, or above the level of the umbilicus for a full-term pregnancy of a breech presentation.	7. To search for the clearest signal (obtained by placing the transducer over the location of the fetal heart at the point of maximum intensity)

Procedure	Rationale
8. Adjust the audio-volume control while moving the transducer over the abdomen.	8. To obtain the loudest audible fetal signal
9. Count the maternal radial pulse.	9. To differentiate between maternal and fetal heart rates
10. Secure the ultrasound transducer with the abdominal belt or other fixation device.	10. To prevent displacement of the transducer
11. Observe the signal-quality indicator.	11. To verify clarity of input based on correct placement of the transducer
12. Set the recorder at a paper speed of 3 cm/min and observe the FHR on the monitor strip. NOTE: A speed of 1 to 2 cm/min is used in some countries.	12. To ensure that the paper feeds correctly and that the recording is clear
13. Depress the test button if the monitor does not self-test when turned on.	13. To verify that the monitor prints out the predetermined number on the corresponding line of the monitor strip according to manufacturer guidelines
14. Check the time printed on the monitor strip (reset monitor clock as necessary). If using a computer documentation system, check that the time correlates with the computer system. If using a paperless system, ensure correct time on monitor screen.	14. To ensure that the monitor prints out or electronically records the accurate time and that data are being captured
15. Observe and document the baseline FHR *between* contractions or periodic changes.	15. To enable future assessment from the baseline tracing
16. Periodically clean the transducer and maternal abdomen with a damp cloth to remove dried gel. Reapply ultrasonic coupling gel as needed.	16. To promote the woman's comfort

Procedure	Rationale
17. Reposition the transducer whenever the fetal signal becomes unclear (e.g., when the woman moves or when the fetus descends in the pelvis).	17. To ensure a clear, interpretable tracing during fetal monitoring
18. Carefully remove the transducer from the fixation device at the completion of monitoring, and cleanse the abdomen of gel.	18. To avoid damage to the transducer and remove accumulated gel from the abdomen
19. Box 3-1 gives guidelines for care, cleaning, and storage of external transducers.	19. To prevent damage and ensure cleanliness of equipment

---

Box 3-1   General Guidelines for Care, Cleaning, and Storage of External Transducers

- Exercise caution when removing and handling the ultrasound and tocotransducers so that they are not dropped or allowed to swing against any equipment, to protect from damage.
- Clean transducers according to the manufacturer's operating manual, usually with a soft cloth using mild soap and water. Avoid submerging transducers or placing them beneath running water. Do not use alcohol or other cleaning solutions that may damage equipment.
- Gently and loosely coil cables for storage. Avoid tight coiling and sharp bending of the cables, which will result in damage to the wires or casing.
- Cables between monitor models and manufacturers are usually not interchangeable. Forced insertion into an incompatible monitor port is likely to result in damage.
- Dispose of disposable abdominal belts. Wash reusable belts according to the facility's or the manufacturer's suggested procedure before the next use.

Advantages and limitations of ultrasound transducer
Advantages

- Noninvasive
- Easy to apply
- May be used during the antepartum period
- May be used with telemetry
- Does not require ruptured membranes or cervical dilatation
- No known hazards to woman or fetus
- Provides continuous recording of FHR
- Provides permanent record of FHR

Limitations

- May limit maternal movement.
- Requires repositioning with fetal or maternal position change that results in loss of signal.
- Can assess only relative short-term variability.
- May double-count a slow FHR of less than 60 bpm (because of the inability to distinguish the first from the second heart sound so that they are both counted as equals); verify count with auscultation.
- May half-count a tachyarrhythmia of more than 180 bpm (because of the inability to reset, which can result in the skipping or elimination of every other heartbeat); verify count with auscultation.
- Maternal heart rate may be counted if the ultrasound transducer is placed over the maternal arterial vessels, such as the aorta.
- Obese women may be difficult to monitor because of the distance between the transducer and the fetal heart.

Tocotransducer
Description

The tocotransducer (toco) monitors uterine activity transabdominally by means of a pressure-sensing button that is depressed by uterine contractions or fetal movement. The uterine activity panel of the monitor paper displays the *relative* frequency and duration of contractions. Intensity and resting tone can be assessed only with the intrauterine catheter or with palpation. The tocotransducer can be used to monitor uterine activity during both antepartum and intrapartum periods.

Placement of tocotransducer

The following chart shows in a sequential format the procedure and rationale for the application of the tocotransducer:

Procedure	Rationale
1. Explain the procedure to the woman and her family.	1. To allay anxiety
2. Gather the necessary equipment: fetal monitor, tocotransducer, and the equipment desired to monitor the FHR.	2. To ensure that all equipment is readily accessible
3. Position the woman in a comfortable semilateral position.	3. To maximize uteroplacental blood flow by avoiding supine hypotension syndrome
4. Perform Leopold's maneuvers (see Figure 3-2).	4. To determine fetal position, lie, and presentation
5. Align and insert the tocotransducer plug into the appropriate monitor port labeled Toco or UA (for uterine activity).	5. To provide connection without damaging connector pins (could result in a faulty signal)
6. Place the transducer on the maternal abdomen over the upper uterine segment where there is the least amount of maternal tissue between the pressure-sensing button and the uterus (where uterine contractions are best palpated).	6. To ensure that the upper uterine segment is as close as possible to the pressure-sensing button
7. Secure the tocotransducer with the abdominal belt and ensure that there is no gel under the tocotransducer.	7. To prevent displacement of the transducer and to ensure that there is no gel accumulation that might impede function
8. Set the recorder at a paper speed of 3 cm/min, check the printed time/date for	8. To ensure that the paper feeds correctly, the date is accurate, and the recording is clear and

Procedure	Rationale
accuracy, and observe the monitor strip or computer screen. NOTE: A speed of 1 to 2 cm/min is used in some countries.	received by the monitoring system
9. Between contractions, press the UA or Toco test button for the resting baseline to print at the 20 mm Hg line on the monitor strip.	9. To prevent missing the very beginning or ending of the uterine contraction (necessary for FHR pattern interpretation)
10. Monitor the frequency and duration of the contractions and document them in the woman's flow chart according to facility policy.	10. The tocotransducer *cannot* measure intensity of contractions or resting tone between contractions because the depression of the pressure-sensing button varies with amount of maternal adipose tissue; therefore the information should not be relied on to assess need for analgesia in relation to perceived strength (painful-ness) of contractions as registered by the monitor
11. When monitoring is in progress, readjust abdominal belt periodically, and massage any reddened skin areas.	11. To promote comfort and maintain the proper position of the transducer
12. Palpate the fundus every 30 to 60 minutes; do not rely on peak of contraction on monitor tracing to determine the need for analgesia or titration of oxytocin.	12. To assess the relative pressure of the contractions, because the tocotransducer can relate only frequency and duration of contrac-tions; it cannot assess intensity of UC or resting tone
13. Reposition the transducer periodically and secure the abdominal belt snugly.	13. To promote and ensure a good recording

Procedure	Rationale
14. Carefully remove the transducer from the fixation device at the completion of monitoring.	14. To avoid damage to the transducer
15. See Box 3-1 for guidelines for care, cleaning, and storage of external transducers.	15. To prevent damage and ensure cleanliness of equipment

Advantages and limitations of tocotransducer

Advantages

- Noninvasive
- Does not require ruptured membranes or cervical dilatation
- Is easily applied
- May be used with telemetry
- Provides continuous recording of contraction frequency and duration

Limitations

- Information limited to frequency and duration
- Cannot assess strength or intensity of contractions
- Periodic repositioning of transducer may be necessary
- Limits woman's mobility
- May not be able to detect uterine contractions or obtain an interpretable tracing from an obese woman

Internal Mode of Monitoring

Spiral Electrode

Description

The spiral electrode monitors the fetal ECG from the presenting part. It can be applied only after the membranes have been ruptured, when the cervix is dilated 2 to 3 cm or more, and when the presenting part is accessible and identifiable (Figure 3-7). Therefore the spiral electrode can be used only during the intrapartum period.

Contraindications

- Planned application to the fetal face, fontanels, or genitalia
- Inability to identify the portion of the fetus where application is contemplated

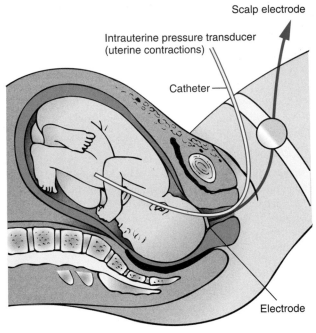

Scalp electrode

Intrauterine pressure transducer
(uterine contractions)

Catheter

Electrode

Figure 3-7
Diagrammatic representation of internal mode of monitoring
with intrauterine catheter and spiral electrode in place.
(From Lowdermilk DL, Perry SE: *Maternity & women's health care,* ed 8,
St Louis, 2004, Mosby.)

- Presence or suspicion of placenta previa
- Presence of active herpes lesions, hepatitis, or HIV infection

Situations requiring caution

- Woman is positive for group B streptococcus, hepatitis B, hepatitis C, syphilis, or gonorrhea
- When the fetus is premature

It is important to refer to the manufacturer's directions and guidelines, and to your own institution's policy and procedures.

Placement of fetal spiral electrode

A licensed registered nurse may insert the spiral electrode but only if this is allowed by licensing board regulations and if the nurse is credentialed and approved by the institution's policies. A sequential format for insertion and use of the spiral electrode is provided in the following chart:

Procedure	Rationale
1. Explain the procedure to the woman and her family.	1. To allay anxiety
2. Gather necessary equipment: gloves, disposable spiral electrode, leg plate interface cable, and attachment pad. Open packaging; remove wires from between drive tube and guide tube.	2. To ensure that all equipment is readily accessible
3. Turn power on and insert cable into the appropriate monitor port, labeled Cardio or ECG.	3. To connect cable plug to appropriate outlet
4a. Assist the health care provider in performing (or perform, if credentialed) a sterile vaginal examination in order to apply the spiral electrode.	4a. To maintain aseptic technique
b. Apply gloves and perform a sterile vaginal examination to determine presenting fetal part.	b. Avoid the fetal face, fontanels, and genitalia
c. Retract spiral electrode until tip is approximately 1 inch into drive handle and introduce into vagina with non-examining hand, keeping examining fingers on target area.	c. To prevent damage to the vaginal wall, glove puncture, and injury to examining fingers during placement
d. Place the guide tube between the examining fingers and place firmly against the target area of the fetus.	d. To ensure proper placement

Procedure	Rationale
e. Rotate the drive and guide tubes clockwise approximately 1½ rotations until resistance is met. Do not continue to rotate the device.	e. To ensure proper depth of placement, and to avoid tissue injury from excessive placement depth
f. Release the electrode wires from the locking device or handle notch and slide the drive and guide tubes off the electrode wires and out of the vagina.	f. To maintain proper placement and safe removal of device
5. Discard the outer drive tube when the application procedure is completed.	5. The electrode must be securely attached to ensure a good signal
6. Connect to the leg plate cable and secure on the woman's thigh.	6. To avoid tension, pulling, or dislodging the spiral electrode
7. Observe the signal quality indicator.	7. To verify clear signal from electrode
8. Set the recorder at a paper speed of 3 cm/min, and observe the FHR on the strip chart. NOTE: A paper speed of 1-2 cm/min is used in some countries.	8. To ensure that the paper feeds correctly and that the recording is clear
9. Check the time printed on the monitor strip and reset monitor clock if necessary.	9. To verify that the monitor records the accurate time
10. Depress the test button if the monitor does not self-test when turned on.	10. To verify that the monitor displays and prints out the predetermined number on the corresponding line of the monitor strip according to the manufacturer's guidelines
11. During monitoring, check the attachment plate periodically, and reposition for comfort as needed.	11. To ensure transmission of the signal

Procedure	Rationale
12. When removing the spiral electrode, turn 1½ rotations counter-clockwise or until it is free from the fetal presenting part. Do not pull the electrode from the fetal skin. Do not cut wires and pull apart to remove electrode from the fetus. Disconnect the electrode from the leg plate, remove the attachment pad, and dispose of the electrode and the attachment pad according to facility policy.	12. To ensure that the electrode is removed in the same manner that it was applied; pulling the electrode straight out results in unnecessary trauma to the fetal skin, produces an observable wound, and predisposes the site to infection
13. The electrode should be removed just before cesarean delivery, vacuum extractor use, and forceps.	13. In cesarean delivery, the electrode should not be left attached and brought up through the uterine incision. If unable to detach, cut wire at perineum and notify physician
14. Clean the leg plate cable, if reusable, according to the facility's procedure, or follow the manu-facturer's directions in the operating manual.	14. To prevent infection
15. Loosely coil the cable and place in a secure area.	15. To prevent damage to the wires (can occur with tight coiling, resulting in loss of or an inadequate fetal signal)
16. Observe the fetal insertion site and cleanse with soap and water if indicated or as directed by policy.	16. To detect or prevent inflammation

Advantages and limitations of spiral electrode
Advantages

- Can assess both long- and short-term variability
- Positional changes do not affect quality of tracing

- Can accurately display some fetal cardiac arrhythmias (if logic switch is off [see later under Artifact Detection]) when linked to ECG recorder
- Accurately displays FHR between 30 and 240 bpm
- Is more comfortable than external transducer belt

Limitations

- Membranes must be ruptured
- Cervix must be dilated at least 2 cm
- Presenting part must be accessible and identifiable
- Need moist environment for FHR detection (difficult to monitor when fetal head is crowning)
- May record maternal heart rate (with fetal demise)
- May miss fetal arrhythmias if logic switch is on
- May not get good conduction when excessive fetal hair is present

Intrauterine Pressure Catheter

Description

The intrauterine pressure catheter or transducer (IUP, IUPC, or IUPT) monitors contraction frequency, duration, intensity, and resting tone (Figure 3-8). A small catheter is introduced vaginally (transcervically) into the uterus after the cervix is dilated 2 to 3 cm or sufficiently to identify the presenting part, and the fetal membranes have been ruptured. The catheter is compressed during uterine contractions, placing pressure on a transducer. The pressure is then reflected on the monitor tracing in units of millimeters of mercury (mm Hg).

Intrauterine pressure catheters that have the pressure-sensing device within the catheter tip or cable do not require an instillation of sterile water for use. These catheters are provided with an amnioport (Intran Plus, Koala, and Saflex) to allow simultaneous amniofusion and uterine activity monitoring. Always refer to the manufacturer's directions and guidelines, along with your facility's policies and procedures, for further information.

Placement of intrauterine pressure catheter

A licensed registered nurse may insert the intrauterine pressure catheter, but only if this is allowed by licensing board regulations and if the nurse is credentialed and approved by the institution's policies. The following chart shows the procedure in a sequential format for the use and insertion of the intrauterine pressure catheter.

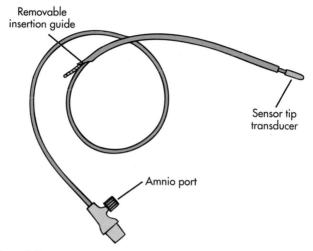

Figure 3-8

Intrauterine catheter with the sensor transducer located in the tip of the catheter provides uninterrupted uterine activity monitoring. Saline-filled catheters are another type of catheter in use. Note that this catheter has an amnioport that may be used for an amnioinfusion.

Procedure	Rationale
1. Explain the procedure to the woman and her family.	1. To allay anxiety
2. Gather necessary equipment: disposable intrauterine kit, sterile gloves, and other equipment to perform a sterile vaginal examination.	2. To ensure that all equipment is readily accessible
3. Turn the power on and insert the reusable cable into the appropriate monitor connector labeled UA, Toco, or Utero.	3. To activate the pressure transducer

Procedure	Rationale
4. Depending on the make of catheter, zero the monitor after connecting to the cable and prior to insertion. Refer to manufacturer's directions for zeroing instructions.	4. To establish a zero baseline for the catheter system based on normal atmospheric pressure
5. If inserting a fluid-filled catheter, fill the catheter with 5 ml sterile water, leaving the syringe attached to the catheter. Maintain sterility at the maternal end of the catheter.	5. To ensure that the catheter is patent and fluid-filled before insertion; to maintain aseptic technique
6a. Prepare the woman and assist with a sterile vaginal examination. Identify the fetal presenting part.	6a. To maintain aseptic technique and to identify the optimal location for catheter insertion
b. Insert the sterile catheter and introducer guide inside the cervix between the examining fingers; do not extend introducer guide beyond fingertips.	b. The guide is made of a hard plastic that can cause trauma if inserted farther than necessary
c. Advance only the catheter according to the insertion depth indicator or until the blue/black or stop mark on it reaches the vaginal introitus.*	c. To ensure that enough of the catheter is inside the uterus (approximately 30 to 45 cm)
d. Separate and remove or slide the catheter introducer guide away from the introitus and remove; dispose of the guide appropriately.	d. To prevent the guide from sliding toward the introitus
7. Secure the catheter to the woman's leg.	7. To ensure the woman's mobility without fear of dislodging the catheter
8. Encourage the woman to cough.	8. To confirm a sharp spike on uterine activity tracing

*Remove catheter immediately in the event of *extraovular* placement outside of the amniotic fluid space (between the chorionic membrane and endometrial lining), as evidenced by blood in the catheter.

Procedure	Rationale
9. Document baseline resting tone in the supine position with left lateral and right lateral tilt.	9. To obtain baseline information, as maternal position and IUPC position may alter measurements
10. Re-zero monitor if indicated during labor, according to manufacturer's directions.	10. To ensure that uterine activity information is correct
11. Gently remove catheter after use and discard; store reusable cable for future use.	11. To ensure that disposable catheter is not reused

Fluid-filled catheters

When monitoring is in progress,

a. Flush the intrauterine catheter with sterile water every 2 hours or as necessary (the use of solutions other than sterile water can occlude and corrode the system)	a. To remove any vernix caseosa or air bubbles that may have entered the catheter and can invalidate the pressure reading
b. Check the proper functioning of the catheter when necessary by tapping the catheter, asking the woman to cough, or applying fundal pressure while observing the chart	b. To ensure inflection on the chart paper, zero the catheter and test according to the manufacturer's directions

Advantages and limitations of intrauterine catheter
Advantages

- Less confining and more comfortable than external mode of uterine activity monitoring
- Only accurate measure of uterine activity (e.g., frequency, duration, intensity, and resting tone)
- Records accurately regardless of maternal position
- Allows for an amnioinfusion to dilute meconium and treat variable decelerations that are uncorrected with other interventions
- Allows calculation of Montevideo units

Limitations

- Membranes must be ruptured and cervix sufficiently dilated (e.g., 2 to 3 cm)
- Improper insertion can cause maternal or placental trauma
- May have an increased risk for infection

A fetal monitoring equipment checklist (Table 3-1) can be used to check for and ensure proper functioning of the equipment. The woman who is electronically monitored should be given, if she expresses interest, an explanation of equipment operations to allay any anxiety. The care given to the electronically monitored woman is the same as that given to any woman during labor, with the additional consideration of those factors that relate directly to the monitor. Guidelines for educating the woman and family about electronic fetal monitoring are provided in the last section of this chapter, and care of the monitored patient is described in Chapter 10.

Display of Fetal Heart Rate, Uterine Activity, and Other Information

The display on the front of the monitor shows the FHR and the uterine pressure, and it identifies the signal source for each (Figure 3-9). Additional monitor options include maternal noninvasive blood pressure (NBP), maternal heart rate, maternal pulse oximetry, maternal pulse rate obtained either by pulse oximetry or by NBP, maternal ECG in real time, gross fetal body movements, and fetal pulse oximetry. These parameters are also displayed on the front or face of the monitor.

Other data, in addition to the FHR and uterine activity, may be printed on the monitor strip. The time of day, date, and paper speed are usually printed every 10 minutes. The signal source is usually printed on every three or four pages of the tracing and with each change of parameter and mode of monitoring. Depending on the monitor's options, other maternal and fetal data may be printed on the tracing. The maternal heart rate and maternal ECG can be trended on the upper (or heart rate) section of the monitor strip. Fetal pulse oximetry values can be continuously printed on the lower (or uterine activity) section of the paper. Some monitors continuously print maternal pulse oximetry values on the lower section of the tracing or print them as whole numbers after each

Table 3-1   Fetal monitoring equipment checklist

Name: _____		Evaluator: _____		
Date: _____				
Items To Be Checked		Yes	No	Remarks

Preparation of Monitor

1. Is the paper inserted correctly?
2. Is the paper speed set for
   3 cm/min speed?
3. Are the transducer cables plugged
   securely into the appropriate port?
4. Verify monitor date/time when using
   electronic documentation.

Ultrasound (US) Transducer

1. Has US transmission gel been applied
   to the transducer?
2. Was the FHR tested and noted on the
   monitor strip?
3. Does a signal light flash or an audible
   beep sound with each heartbeat?
4. Is the belt secure and snug but
   comfortable?

Tocotransducer

1. Is the tocotransducer firmly positioned
   where there is the least maternal
   tissue?
2. Has the tocotransducer been applied
   without gel or paste?
3. Was the UA reference depressed
   between contractions?
4. Is the belt secure and snug?

Spiral Electrode

1. Are the wires inserted correctly into
   the leg plate?
2. Is the spiral electrode attached to the
   presenting part of the fetus?
3. Is the pre-gelled electrode pad
   secured to mother's leg or abdomen?

Continued

Table 3-1   Fetal monitoring equipment checklist—cont'd

Items To Be Checked	Yes	No	Remarks
Intrauterine Pressure Catheter (IUPC)			
1. Is the length line on the catheter visible at the introitus?			
2. Is it noted on the monitor paper that a test or calibration was done?			
3. Has the monitor been set to zero according to the manufacturer's directions?			
4. Is the IUPC properly secured to the patient?			
5. Is baseline resting tone of uterus documented?			

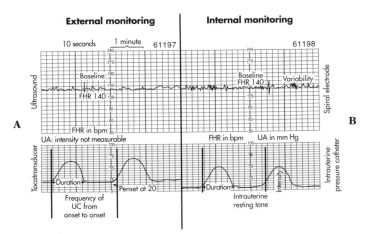

Figure 3-9
Display of fetal heart rate and uterine activity on monitor strips.
A, External mode of monitoring with ultrasound and tocotransducer as the signal source. **B,** Internal mode of monitoring with spiral electrode and intrauterine catheter as the signal source. Frequency of uterine contractions are measured from the onset of one contraction to the onset of the next.

measurement. Maternal NBP can also be printed as whole numbers. The manufacturer's operating manual should be available and referred to for more information, especially when assessing women with risk factors who may have concurrent monitoring of multiple parameters.

Monitor tracing scale

The FHR and uterine activity (UA) are printed on scaled paper. The FHR is printed on the upper section and the uterine activity on the lower section. Monitors are preset by their manufacturers for the countries in which they are used. Note the differences in the range and scale of the fetal heart rate and uterine activity sections, as well as in the paper/recorder speed, in Figure 3-10. The monitor strip in Figure 3-10, *A*, depicts the tracing paper that is used with monitors used in North America, with a speed of 3 cm/min. The monitor strip in Figure 3-10, *B*, depicts the tracing paper that is used in many countries outside North America, with a speed of 1 cm/min.

It is imperative to use paper that is correctly scaled to match the domestic (3 cm/min) or international (1 cm/min) monitor settings. For example, if paper scaled for North America is used and the monitor is set for international use, the FHR baseline rate will visually widen and the height and depth of periodic changes will visually increase.

Monitoring twins and multiples

Many monitors have the capability of monitoring twin gestations at the same time. Monitoring of twins may be done with two separate ultrasound transducers, or one fetus may be monitored by direct fetal scalp electrode (Figure 3-11). The dual tracings may be distinguished by a thicker or darker trace for one fetus and a thinner or lighter trace for the other fetus (see Figure 3-6). Another option to distinguish the tracings between twins is a "twin offset" mechanism, which separates the two fetal heart rates on the tracing by a distance of about 20 bpm. Thus one twin appears to have an FHR that is higher than the actual heart rate. The manufacturer's instruction manual should be consulted to have a clear understanding of this capability.

To clearly differentiate between twins, their positions in the uterus can be documented and ultrasound transducers labeled. In identifying twins or multiples, the fetus in the advanced position

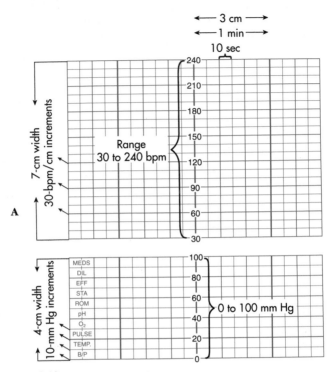

Figure 3-10
A, Fetal monitor paper scale: 3 cm/min speed used in North America.

Vertical Axis
Heart Rate
Range   30 to 240 beats per minute (bpm)
Scale   Increments of 30 bpm/cm
Uterine Activity
Range   0-100 mm Hg pressure
Scale   Increments of 5 or 10 mm Hg
Horizontal Axis
Paper/recorder speed   3 cm/min = six 10-second subsections
                         within 1 minute

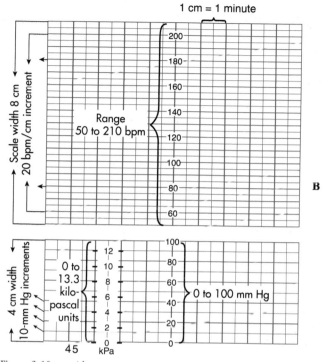

Figure 3-10, cont'd

B, Fetal monitor paper scale: 1 cm per min speed used in countries outside North America, with key points identified.

Vertical Axis

Heart Rate

Range   50 to 210 bpm

Scale   Increments of 20 bpm/cm

Uterine Activity

Range   0-100 mm Hg pressure, or 0 to
                     13.3 kilopascal units (1 kPa = 7.5 mm Hg)

Scale   Increments of 10 mm Hg

Horizontal Axis

Paper/recorder speed   1 cm/min = two subsections
                        (or 2 cm/min speed = four
                        subsections)

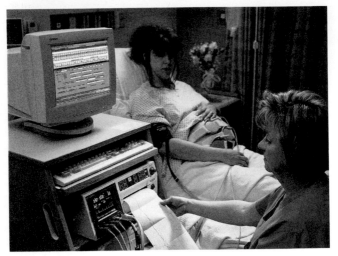

Figure 3-11
Monitoring of twin gestation with two separate ultrasound transducers.
(Courtesy GE Medical Systems Information Technologies, Milwaukee, Wis.)

just above the cervix is labeled A, the next one B, and so on. Monitoring three or more fetuses is very difficult, but in the case of triplets, where the C triplet is the furthest from the cervix, monitoring may be achieved with two monitors. In doing this, however, it is important to place the second toco adjacent to the first one, in order to evaluate the FHR on the basis of the uterine contraction (Murray, 1997).

The cross-channel verification alert may occur if both fetuses have the same/coincident heart rates. If this occurs, relocate the tocotransducer(s) to detect the second FHR.

The Fetal Monitor, Systems, and the Woman

Artifact Detection

Fetal monitors have built-in artifact rejection systems, which are always in operation when using the external mode of FHR monitoring. Logic circuitry rejects data when there is a greater variation than is expected between successive fetal heartbeats. When repetitive variations vary by more than the accepted amount, newer monitors continue to print regardless of the extent of the excursion of the FHR.

The older-generation monitors may switch from a hold mode to a non-record mode. The recorder resumes recording when the variations between successive beats fall within the predetermined parameters.

During internal monitoring, artifact is rare, and the logic system will miss only those changes that exceed the predetermined limits of the system. If there is an accessible switch to select a logic or no-logic mode, it is preferable to have the monitor in the no-logic mode when using the internal mode (spiral electrode) to detect fetal arrhythmias. When recording internally, the logic-on mode should be used only when there is true artifact, such as when there is a low signal-to-noise ratio (caused by extraneous electrical noise), or when there is a large maternal R wave that is counted on an intermittent basis. This can usually be determined by printing out the fetal ECG.

Troubleshooting the Monitor

The electronic fetal monitor is a useful tool to assess fetal well-being. As with any electronic device, problems may occur, but they can often be overcome. A fetal monitoring equipment checklist (Table 3-1) can be used to screen for appropriate application of the monitor. The following chart suggests actions for identified electro-mechanical problems.

Problem	Action
Power	■ Check power cord at wall and back of monitor.
Ultrasound	
Half or double rate	■ Assess FHR with fetoscope, stethoscope, or Doppler.
	■ Check maternal pulse to rule out maternal signal, and document maternal pulse.
	■ Reapply ultrasound gel and recheck.
	■ Move transducer to search for a better signal.
	■ Consider applying spiral electrode.

Problem	Action
Erratic trace or display	■ Reposition transducer. ■ Reposition woman. ■ Tighten ultrasound belt if too loose. ■ Check gel on transducer (if it is dry, sound waves do not penetrate the skin). Reapply gel if needed. Move transducer if fetus is out of range.

Spiral electrode

Problem	Action
Erratic trace or display	■ Use a new spiral electrode. ■ Check that reference electrode is in vaginal secretions (instill fluid if necessary). ■ Check attachment pad on leg for adherence to skin. ■ Ensure that connection of electrode is secure on attachment pad and that connector is securely inserted into the leg-plate cable.
Signal quality indicator is continuously red	■ Ensure that logic switch is off to assess for fetal arrhythmia.

Tocotransducer

Problem	Action
Not recording	■ Check that cable is plugged into monitor and power is on.
Numbers in high range	■ Readjust toco on abdomen; ensure that cable is fully attached to monitor. ■ Zero monitor with toco/UA button between contractions, or replace with another toco.
Toco not picking up contractions	■ Palpate abdomen for best location to sense contractions, and reapply toco.

Problem	Action
Toco not picking up contractions—cont'd	■ Test toco by depressing pressure transducer and observing readout on monitor.
	■ Tighten belt, or use another device to hold toco firmly against abdomen.
	■ Consider using intrauterine pressure catheter (IUPC) if the woman is significantly obese.
Intrauterine pressure catheter	
Not recording	■ Recheck cable insertion.
	■ Flush fluid-filled catheter.
Resting tone (>25 mm Hg)	■ Palpate abdomen to identify uterine tonus before making equipment adjustments.
	■ Adjust level of strain gauge for fluid-filled catheters to maternal xypoid.
	■ Zero or recalibrate non–fluid-filled catheter.
	■ Flush fluid-filled catheter.
Not recording contractions	■ Check catheter markings at woman's introitus (catheter may have slipped out).
	■ Replace catheter if necessary.
High resting tone	■ Higher resting tone may be noted with multiple gestation, uterine malformation or fibroids, use of oxytocin, amnioinfusion, extraovular placement.
	■ Decrease or discontinue oxytocin or amnioinfusion in presence of uterine hypertonus.
	■ Re-zero monitor.
	■ Replace catheter if incorrect placement.

Problem	Action
Potential problems	
Fetal arrhythmia	■ Auscultate FHR with fetoscope or stethoscope. ■ Check for tachycardia or bradycardia. ■ Perform fetal ECG.
Errors caused by incorrect paper speed or paper with different scale	■ Check annotation with paper speed: it should be 3 cm/min in North America. ■ Check scale: it should be 30 to 240 bpm for FHR if paper speed is 3 cm/min, or 50 to 210 bpm if paper speed is 1 or 2 cm/min.
Cross-channel verification alert	■ Alert occurs with two coincidental heart rates. Verify maternal heart rate. Reposition ultrasound transducer(s) to detect second fetal heart rate.

Telemetry

Remote internal or external FHR monitoring via radio wave telemetry (Figure 3-12) helps women remain ambulatory without the loss of continuous monitoring data. A woman may feel less confined, more relaxed, and more content if she can walk around. The transducer is worn by means of an abdominal belt or other device (Figure 3-13). Heart rate and uterine activity signals are continuously transmitted to a receiver that is connected to the fetal monitor. The monitor then processes and displays the data, and it prints the heart rate and uterine activity on the monitor strip. The telemetry unit should be connected to a fetal monitor that is hard-wired to the central display to enable surveillance by clinicians.

In addition to standard ultrasound and tocotransducers, external watertight transducers are available. These can be used to continue fetal surveillance under water. For example, a woman can use a watertight transducer with a wireless telemetry device when in a shower, spa, or bathtub.

In addition to providing the benefits of freedom of movement during labor and continuous monitoring in the labor suite or the

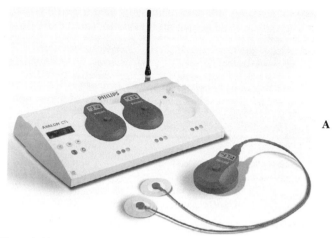

A

Figure 3-12
A, The cordless transducer system (Avalon CTS) combines
fetal monitoring technology with radiofrequency (telemetry)
technology. This system eliminates the need for cables.
Waterproof transducers may be used for the patient who is in
bed, ambulating, or in the bath.
(Courtesy Philips Medical Systems, Böhlingen, Germany.)

delivery room, telemetry has been applied in the outpatient setting
for women instructed to remain at rest in their own homes. Data
from the transmitter can be sent via modem to the receiver unit,
which is connected to a printer, producing a hard copy of the FHR
monitor strip. This transmission of information from the woman to
the receiver unit allows the clinician to determine the woman's
status. With the data received, the clinician can adjust the woman's
care and can also consult with a referral center and receive an
expert's interpretation of the data.

Central Display

A central monitor display at the nurses' station provides an opportunity to view tracings from several women at the same time
(Figure 3-14). Single-screen displays of several women or of one
woman can be accessed from remote locations, including the

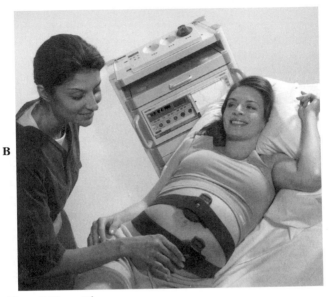

Figure 3-12, cont'd
B, Cordless transducers are applied to the maternal abdomen for external monitoring. The base station above the fetal monitor is compatible with Philips (formerly HP) Series 50 fetal monitors. An automated frequency search at the base station prevents confusion of transducers with multiple systems.
(Courtesy Philips Medical Systems, Böblingen, Germany.)

bedside, the staff locker room or lounge area, the physician's office, or at home. Thus the staff can have instant access to the monitor patterns from many locations, which is especially important when the nurse cannot be in constant attendance. Some systems include the capability of data entry in the form of detailed notes about examination results, cervical dilatation, fetal station, administration of drugs, the woman's position, and vital signs, all related to time. Reports can even be generated with a printer linked to the display, which can provide a single and comprehensive document containing information, history, and a graphic printout of the labor curve progression.

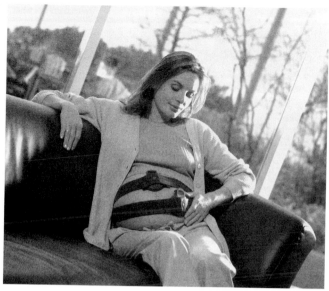

Figure 3-13
The cordless transducer system allows the woman mobility, providing a choice of positions while the fetus is being monitored.
(Courtesy Philips Medical Systems, Böblingen, Germany.)

Some central display systems (Figure 3-15) can provide additional information, including the following:

- A *system status* screen provides an instant overview of several beds on the system and indicates any alerts by room number. In addition, it can identify the signal source of any woman on the system.
- A *trend screen* can provide the most recent few minutes of heart rate and uterine activity data on any one woman, with immediate warning of critical conditions relating to any woman in the system.
- An *alert screen* can provide an immediate summary of the trend analysis on any woman. The data can be made available to the staff before, during, and after an alert.

Computer-Based Information Systems

Information systems combine fetal surveillance and alerting with documentation and data storage into one system that can cover the

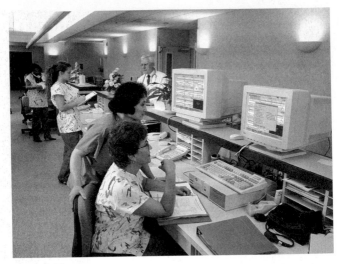

Figure 3-14
Patient care staff at a central station monitoring a number of women.
(Courtesy GE Medical Systems Information Technologies, Milwaukee, Wis. Photograph by Jim Fiora.)

entire continuum of obstetrical care across several pregnancies. The surveillance component of the system can be set to alert for fetal tachycardia or bradycardia, signal loss, coincidental fetal and maternal heart rates, and other parameters. Ranges for the duration of, and recovery from, fetal bradycardia or tachycardia can be set at different levels for each woman. These systems are available from some of the companies that manufacture fetal monitors as well as other companies such as Hill-Rom with the Watch Child system (Batesville, Ind.).

In addition to improving the quality of care through surveillance and alert capabilities, a system that is accessible across the health care continuum can also provide a database for statistical reporting for administration, research, and quality purposes, especially when integrated with other hospital or outpatient information systems. Such a system can provide multiple data entry points across the continuum of care and on the various campuses of a hospital network (Kelly, 1999). These points include the physician's

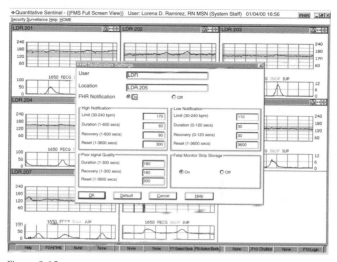

Figure 3-15

The surveillance system provides an overview of many women. It also allows the user to set the high/low ranges that will initiate an audible or visual notification of fetal bradycardia and tachycardia. If the heart rate violates the set limits and duration, the notification will continue until it has been acknowledged, even if the heart rate returns to an acceptable level. High/low ranges may be set at different levels for each woman.

(Courtesy GE Medical Systems Information Technologies, Milwaukee, Wis.)

office (Figure 3-16), ambulatory care clinic, antepartum testing center, inpatient department, labor and delivery suite or birthing center, and home health or continuing care department. For example, if a woman presents to the birthing center in the middle of the night, the staff can readily access the entire antenatal record, the home uterine monitoring documents, and the ultrasound, nonstress test, and biophysical profile that were completed just the previous afternoon, even at a different campus within the system.

Documentation on forms and flow sheets together with annotated tracings can quickly and easily provide complete electronic patient records. The *archival* and *retrieval* of the original fetal monitoring strip has proved to be a problem for most medical record departments because the process is labor intensive and the paper is space consuming. Microfiche records are less bulky to

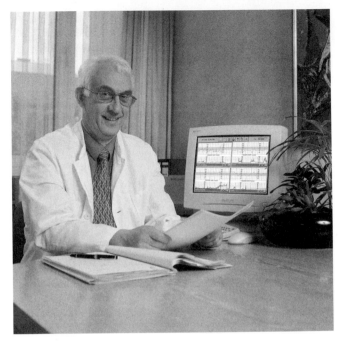

Figure 3-16
The physician can access a fetal heart rate tracing in the
medical office.
(Courtesy Philips Medical Systems, Böblingen, Germany.)

store but still take time to log, sort, and file in the medical record,
although many facilities continue to do this. A welcome alternative
has been computer-based storage systems on the hard drive and
optical laser disks. These systems are best installed with a security
system that prevents alteration or removal of the documents, and
a backup system in the event that there is damage or loss of the
optical disk cartridge.

The ability to have multiple points of data entry, information
retrieval, and reproduction of a woman's record and fetal
monitor tracing is a significant advancement. This, coupled with an
interface to the hospital admission, discharge, and transfer (ADT)
information system and other hospital-based information systems,
should contribute to the trend toward comprehensive, paperless,
and fully electronic information systems.

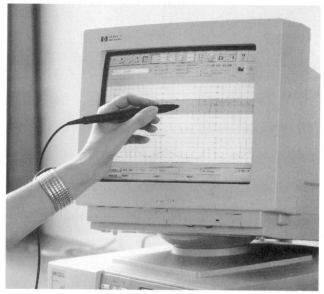

Figure 3-17
With color icons, one can enter and access information
quickly and easily with a light-pen, mouse, or keyboard.
(Courtesy Philips Medical Systems, Böblingen, Germany.)

Data-input devices

Data-input devices can be used with electronic fetal monitors and
monitoring systems. Some of their options include use of a bar-
code reader, keypads for data entry, light-pens (Figure 3-17), touch
screens, remote event markers, and standard keyboards. The input
is subsequently printed on the tracing (Figure 3-18). The use of
these options can promote accurate documentation and help eliminate the need for handwritten annotations, which are sometimes
illegible. Additional information may be entered on the monitor
strip automatically, such as the time, date, paper speed, and signal
source.

Considerations Related to Monitor Purchase

Various monitors are available, and generally they have the same
capabilities. In considering a monitor for purchase, however, it is

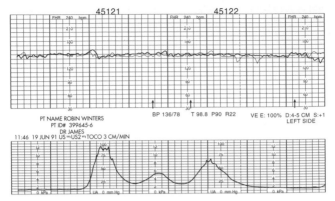

Figure 3-18
Tracing demonstrates pertinent data that have been entered via a data-input device. Note the dual fetal heart rate tracings of twins.
(Courtesy GE Medical Systems Information Technologies, Milwaukee, Wis.)

prudent to use one on a trial basis and to consult with people who have used the type of equipment being considered (Figures 3-19 and 3-20). The following points should also be considered:

1. Accuracy of data output
2. Ease of use
3. Reliability for continuous functioning with minimum downtime for repair
4. Repair frequency and history from other facilities using the same monitor (e.g., turnaround time for service)
5. Cost of monitor and other expendable supplies (e.g., paper, abdominal belts)
6. Availability of expendable supplies from multiple sources for better cost advantage
7. Legible display and function labels
8. Complexity of paper refill procedure
9. Training time needed for users, or video training films included with purchase
10. Training services and support from the company at little or no cost
11. Fragility of ultrasound transducer, cable, and connectors
12. History and stability of company and frequency of changing models

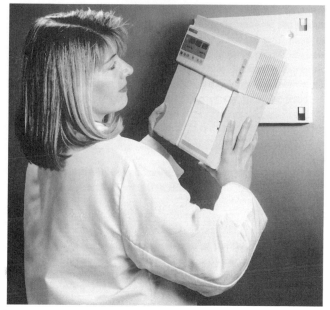

Figure 3-19
The space-saving Series 50 A and IP fetal monitors are compact and lightweight and function equally well mounted on a wall or on a table or mobile cart.
(Courtesy Philips Medical Systems, Böblingen, Germany.)

13. Expected life of the equipment
14. Interchangeability of transducers from one model to the next within the same company (to avoid the possibility of built-in obsolescence)
15. Cost of extended service agreement or warranty

Educating the Woman and Family

The nurse's role is to ensure that the woman and her family understand the instrumentation involved in fetal monitoring and, more especially, how its use can be helpful to them. The following points may be taught, as appropriate:

- Use of the monitor does not imply fetal compromise.
- Fetal monitoring helps to assess fetal well-being and oxygen status.

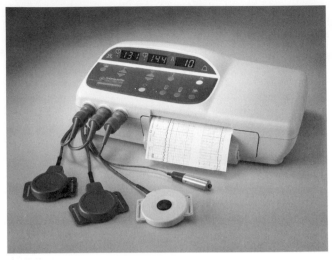

Figure 3-20
The Corometrics 170 Series noninvasive fetal monitor is a compact, lightweight unit with single or dual ultrasound that can be used in the office, clinic, or hospital setting. This monitor features a high/low heart rate alarm, telemetry interface, fetal movement detection capability, and a fetal acoustic stimulator (FASt) interface.
(Courtesy GE Medical Systems Information Technologies, Milwaukee, Wis. Photograph by Jim Fiora.)

- Fetal status via FHR can be continuously assessed even during contractions.
- Lower panel on the monitor strip shows uterine activity and the upper panel shows FHR.
- The volume of the FHR monitor can be turned up or down.
- The FHR sound may not be audible or the tracing not visible for short periods of time because of fetal or maternal movement.
- When using the external tocotransducer, the numbers on the uterine activity panel do not reflect the actual intensity of the contraction.
- The paper speed on the monitor is a reflection of time (e.g., 3 cm/min speed is 1 minute of time; 1 cm/min speed is 1 minute of time; show where the vertical lines reflect the time frame).

- If there is a bedside electronic documentation or central surveillance system, explain how you will be using it; show the woman which display is her fetal monitor tracing and how her labor can be monitored by staff when no one is physically present in the room.
- Prepared childbirth techniques can be implemented without difficulty.
- Effleurage performed during external monitoring can be done on the sides of the abdomen or upper thighs.
- Breathing patterns based on timing and intensity of contractions can be enhanced by observation of the uterine activity panel on the monitor strip but should not take the place of maternal observation.
- Note the peak of a contraction; knowing that the contraction may not get any stronger and is half over can be helpful.
- Note the diminishing intensity of the contraction to see that the contraction is almost over.
- Use of internal modes of monitoring does not have to restrict the woman's movement.
- Use of external modes of monitoring may require the woman's cooperation in positioning and movement.

The woman and her support person should also be made aware that two other factors have an effect on the fetus regardless of the assessment technique: maternal positioning and the Valsalva maneuver (Lowdermilk, Perry, 2004). The lateral position is encouraged to avoid *supine hypotension* syndrome, which occurs when the woman is in the supine position with the weight and pressure of the gravid uterus on the ascending vena cava. This pressure decreases venous return and maternal cardiac output, and it may subsequently cause hypotension. In turn, the intervillous space blood flow is decreased and the resulting hypoxemia may be demonstrated by a nonreassuring FHR pattern.

The *Valsalva maneuver* can occur as the woman holds her breath and bears down during a uterine contraction. This process stimulates the vagus nerve, which decreases the maternal heart rate and blood pressure. Open-glottis breathing is preferred in the second stage of labor when the woman is pushing. This can be achieved by allowing air to escape from the lungs during the pushing process. An audible grunting sound may be heard.

References

American Academy of Pediatrics (AAP), American College of Obstetricians and Gynecologists (ACOG): *Guidelines for perinatal care,* ed 5, Washington, DC, 2002, The Academy and the College.

Association of Women's Health, Obstetric, and Neonatal Nurses (AWHONN): *Fetal heart monitoring: Principles and practices,* ed 3, Dubuque, Iowa, 2003, Kendall/Hunt.

Clinical Effectiveness Support Unit: The use of electronic fetal monitoring: The use and interpretation of cardiotocography in intrapartum fetal surveillance, *Evidence-based Clinical Guideline* no. 8, United Kingdom, 2001, Royal College of Obstetricians and Gynaecologists.

Feinstein NF, Sprague A, Trepanier MJ: Fetal heart rate auscultation: Comparing auscultation to electronic fetal monitoring, *Lifelines* 4(3): 35-44, 2000.

Fraser DM, Cooper MA, editors: *Myles textbook for midwives,* ed 14, London, 2003, Churchill Livingstone.

Freeman RK, Garite TJ, Nageotte MP: *Fetal heart rate monitoring,* Baltimore, 2003, Williams & Wilkins.

Kelly CS: Perinatal computerized patient record and archiving systems: Pitfalls and enhancements for implementing a successful computerized medical record, *J Perinat Neonatal Nurs* 12(4):1-14, 1999.

Lowdermilk DL, Perry SE: *Maternity & women's health care,* ed 8, St Louis, 2004, Mosby.

Murry ML: *Antepartal and intrapartal fetal monitoring,* Albuquerque, NM, 1997, Learning Resources International.

Society of Obstetricians and Gynecologists of Canada (SOGC): Policy statement: Fetal health surveillance in labour, *J SOGC* 24(3):250-276, 2002.

Vintzileos AM, Nochimson DJ, Guzman ER, et al: Intrapartum electronic fetal heart rate monitoring versus intermittent auscultation: A meta-analysis, *Obstet Gynecol* 85(1):149-155, 1995.

Uterine Activity

4

Methods: Palpation and Electronic Monitoring

Assessment of uterine activity (UA) includes the identification of contraction frequency, duration, strength or intensity, and resting tone. Uterine activity can be assessed by manual palpation or by electronic monitoring with either external monitoring using a tocotransducer or an internal intrauterine pressure catheter (IUPC) (Figure 4-1). It is important to have a good understanding of uterine activity and contractions to identify dysfunctional labor patterns that delay or arrest the progress of labor, to identify uterine hyperactivity, to evaluate the fetal heart rate (FHR) in relationship to the uterine contractions, and to provide appropriate support for the woman in labor.

Palpation

Manual palpation is the traditional method of monitoring contractions. This method can measure contraction frequency, duration, and relative strength. Palpation is a learned skill that is best performed with the fingertips to feel the uterus rise upward as the contraction develops. *Mild, moderate,* and *strong* are the terms used to describe the strength of uterine contractions as determined by the examiner's hands during palpation and based on the degree of indentation of the abdomen (AWHONN, 2003). For learning and for the purpose of comparison, the degree of indentation corresponds to the palpation sensation when feeling the parts of the adult face, as described in the following chart:

Contraction Strength	Palpation Sensation
Mild	Tense fundus but easy to indent (feels like touching finger to tip of nose)

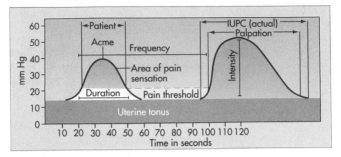

Figure 4-1
Comparison of relative sensitivities of assessing uterine contractions by internal monitoring (IUPC), manual palpation, and patient perception. Note that the woman does not usually perceive the contraction until the uterine pressure increases above the baseline. External monitor is variable.
(Modified from Dickason EJ, Silverman BL, Kaplan JA: *Maternal-infant nursing care,* ed 3, St Louis, 1998, Mosby.)

Contraction Strength	Palpation Sensation
Moderate	Firm fundus, difficult to indent with fingertips (feels like touching finger to chin)
Strong	Rigid, boardlike fundus, almost impossible to indent (feels like touching finger to forehead)

The majority of labors in the world are managed by palpation, which promotes maternal ambulation and freedom of movement. Palpation as the sole method of monitoring uterine activity is less frequent in hospitals in North America than in other countries.

Electronic Monitoring

Electronic monitoring provides continuous data and a permanent record of uterine activity. *External uterine activity monitoring* is achieved using a tocotransducer to provide information about uterine contraction frequency and duration and an idea of relative strength. The electronic display of a contraction depends on the depression of a pressure-sensing device placed on the maternal abdomen, and factors such as where the device is placed and the amount of maternal adipose tissue result in variations of depression. For example, a thin woman may exhibit large inflections when having mild contractions, in contrast to an obese woman, who may exhibit minor inflections when having strong contractions. In addition, belt tightness, position of the tocotransducer, and maternal and fetal position can all greatly affect the recording of uterine activity. Therefore the strength of the uterine contraction must be assessed by manual palpation when uterine activity is externally monitored.

Internal uterine activity monitoring is achieved using an intrauterine pressure catheter that measures absolute intensity of the uterine contraction and resting tone in addition to contraction frequency and duration. The following chart contrasts the data obtained with these two modes of monitoring:

External Mode	Internal Mode
Tocotransducer	**Intrauterine pressure catheter**
Frequency of contractions	
Measured from the onset of one contraction to the onset of the next contraction	Measured from the onset of one contraction to the onset of the next contraction
Duration of contractions	
From beginning to end	From beginning to end
Relative strength/intensity of contractions	
Relative strength depends on abdominal pressure against the pressure-sensing device. The abdomen must be palpated to assess the strength of the contraction based on the degree of indentation of the fundus.	Intensity of contractions measured as the pressure (in mm Hg) at the peak of the contraction
Resting tone	
The abdomen must be palpated to assess resting tone based on degree of indentation of the fundus.	Pressure (mm Hg) between contractions

Electronic display of uterine activity

Uterine activity is monitored and recorded on the lower section of the monitor strip (Figure 4-2). The range of the scale is from 0 to 100 mm Hg pressure. There are five major vertical sections of 20 mm Hg each, and each of the smaller lines in between represents 10 mm Hg. Some tracing paper manufactured in North America has four major vertical sections of 25 mm Hg each, with the smaller lines representing 5 mm Hg pressure in the uterine activity section.

In addition to the display of uterine activity on the monitor strip, there is a digital display on the front of the monitor. The number is higher during uterine contractions and lower during the resting period between contractions. When the woman's uterine activity is being monitored with a tocotransducer, this display is not a quantitation of uterine activity because the pressure-sensing device on the maternal abdomen cannot measure intensity of uterine contractions.

Progression and Quantitation of Labor

The first stage of labor, from the onset of contractions to complete dilatation of the cervix, is divided into two phases, latent and active. Contractions are infrequent and irregular in the latent stage and the woman experiences modest discomfort. Effacement or thinning of the cervix occurs during this phase. During the active phase of labor, the rate of cervical dilation increases and the fetal presenting part descends. This can be visualized on a labor curve, also called a partogram or cervicograph, and it can be used to graph the progress of labor, providing a visual means of recording cervical dilatation and station across the course of time (Figure 4-3). As the fetal presenting part descends and cervical dilatation increases, the lines cross each other in an X pattern. When the woman's progress through the latent and active phases of labor is compared with a normal labor curve, her labor may be identified as normal, dysfunctional, or precipitous.

In addition to using a labor curve to monitor the progress of labor, Montevideo units (MVUs) have been used as a quantitation measure of uterine activity. Calculation of MVUs requires the use of an intrauterine pressure catheter. This method was described by Caldeyro-Barcia in 1957 as the product of the average

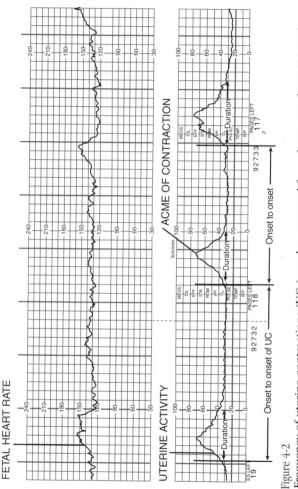

Figure 4-2
Frequency of uterine contractions (UCs) can be measured from the onset of one UC to the onset of the next. Note other identifying information.

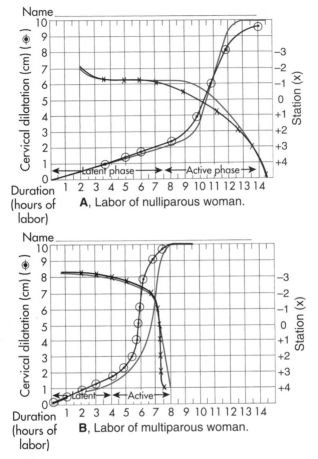

Figure 4-3
Partogram for assessment of patterns of cervical dilatation
and descent. Individual woman's labor patterns *(black)*
superimposed on prepared labor graph for comparison.
A, Labor of a nulliparous woman. **B,** Labor of a multiparous
woman. The rate of cervical dilatation is plotted with the
circled plot points. A line drawn through these symbols
depicts the slope of the curve. Station is plotted with Xs.
A line drawn through the Xs reveals the pattern of descent.
(Modified from Lowdermilk DL, Perry SE: *Maternity & women's health care,* ed 8,
St Louis, 2004, Mosby.)

contraction peak in millimeters of mercury (mm Hg) multiplied by the number of contractions in a 10-minute period (Caldeyro-Barcia, Poseiro, 1960). Another method of calculating MVUs is to subtract the baseline intrauterine pressure (the resting tone) from the peak of the contraction pressure for each contraction in a 10-minute window. These numbers are then added together to determine the number of MVUs. However, in clinical use the value is quickly and roughly obtained by adding the peak intensities of each contraction in a 10-minute period (Parer, 1997). Adequate uterine activity in labor is defined as greater than 200 MVUs. Although investigators have used this quantitation measure, it is limited by not including the duration of the contraction in the calculations.

Normal Uterine Activity

In a normal labor, uterine contractions occur about every 2 to 5 minutes, with a duration of 30 to 60 seconds and an increasing strength from mild to moderate to strong over the course of the labor. Labor patterns vary among individuals (Figure 4-4). When monitored internally, the intensity of the contractions can range from 30 to 80 mm Hg pressure, with a resting tone of less than 20 mm Hg. In addition to providing this information, the monitor strip may also indicate fetal movement by "blips," spikes, or momentary increases in uterine pressure. Accelerations that occur concurrently with fetal movement are a reassuring sign.

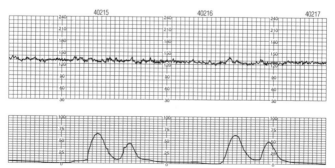

Figure 4-4
Coupling of uterine contractions.

The following chart gives a summary of normal uterine activity patterns.

Frequency   More than 2 minutes between contractions

Duration   Contractions of 30 to 60 seconds (less than 90 seconds)

Intensity   Less than 80 mm Hg pressure (in the first stage of labor)

Resting tone   Thirty seconds or more between contractions; resting intrauterine pressure less than 20 mm Hg (can be determined only by intrauterine monitoring)

Dysfunctional or Abnormal Labor Pattern

A dysfunctional or abnormal labor pattern is one in which labor is slower than normal (protraction disorder), or in which there is a complete cessation of progress (arrest disorder). These terms cannot be applied to the woman who is in the latent stage of labor even if it is prolonged. It is inappropriate to use the terms *dysfunctional* or *abnormal* labor, or to designate *failure to progress,* until the woman has entered the active phase of labor and an adequate trial of labor has been achieved. These terms can be used for the laboring pattern only after an adequate trial of labor and when the diagnostic criteria in the following chart are met (ACOG, 2003).

Labor Pattern	Nulligravida	Multipara
Protraction Disorders		
Dilatation	<1.2 cm/hr	<1.5 cm/hr
Descent	<1.0 cm/hr	<2.0 cm/hr
Arrest Disorders		
Dilatation	>2 hr	>2 hr
Descent	>1 hr	>1 hr

When assessing the uterine activity pattern, the health care provider considers the contraction pattern in terms of frequency, duration, and intensity. MVUs can be assessed for the woman who has an internal intrauterine pressure catheter/transducer. Generally, a good contraction frequency, duration, and intensity, with MVUs exceeding 200 for 2 hours without cervical change, are indicative of an ineffective laboring pattern. Consideration is given to the augmentation of uterine hypocontractility with an oxytocic. Before attributing dystocia to a pelvic problem, inefficient uterine action should be corrected (ACOG, 2003).

Increased Uterine Activity

During intrapartum monitoring of uterine activity, it is important to look for hyperactivity of the uterus in addition to noting the frequency, duration, and intensity of contractions and intrauterine resting tone. Hyperactivity, as evidenced by increased uterine activity on the monitor strip, can result in a decrease in fetal oxygenation because of interference with the uteroplacental circulation. There are varying descriptions and definitions of atypical occurrences related to uterine activity in the literature. Some authors use the terms *tachysystole* and *hyperstimulation* interchangeably; others differentiate them by their effect on the fetal heart rate (ACOG, 1999a). Each institution should develop and utilize appropriate terms and definitions in policies and procedures that are agreed on and substantiated by research.

The following chart defines the terms *hypertonus, tachysystole,* and *hyperstimulation.*

Hypertonus	Abnormally high uterine resting tone (>25 mm Hg pressure) or Montevideo units (>400) (AWHONN, 2003; Freeman et al, 2003)
Tachysystole	Six or more uterine contractions in 10 minutes in consecutive 10-minute intervals (ACOG, 1999a,b); without FHR changes (ACOG, 2003)
Hyperstimulation	Persistent pattern of tachysystole, single contractions lasting >2 minutes, or uterine contractions of normal duration occurring within 1 minute of each other, with demonstrated fetal intolerance (ACOG, 1999a; 2003)

Observations indicating increased uterine activity

- Contractions lasting longer than 90 seconds
- Relaxation lasting less than 30 seconds between contractions
- Inadequate intrauterine relaxation with resting tone greater than 25 mm Hg between contractions
- Peak pressure of contractions greater than 80 mm Hg (without pushing), in the first stage of labor

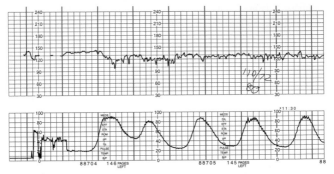

Figure 4-5
Uterine tachysystole. This pattern was noted upon initiation of monitoring. The woman had a transverse fetal lie and a closed cervix and was delivered by primary cesarean for a suspected and then confirmed placental abruption.

- Contractions more frequent than every 2 minutes, or six or more contractions in a 10-minute window in consecutive 10-minute intervals (Figure 4-5)
- Montevideo units greater than 400

Causes of increased uterine activity

- Oxytocin infusion for induction or augmentation of labor
- Oxytocics other than oxytocin (e.g., prostaglandins)
- Abruptio placentae
- Uterine overdistension from amnioinfusion
- Overdistension of the uterine wall as a result of multiple gestation, hydramnios, or a macrosomic fetus
- Pregnancy-induced hypertension
- Drugs: acetylcholine, ergonovine, estrogen, norepinephrine, oxytocin, propranolol, prostaglandins, quinine, sparteine sulfate, vasopressin (Freeman et al, 2003)

Clinical significance

Uterine hyperstimulation, which is generally considered to be iatrogenic, describes a reaction of the myometrium to exogenous oxytocics. This includes oxytocin and prostaglandins to which the myometrium is hypersensitive, or an excessive dose of the drug (McKenzie, 1999) (Figure 4-6). The fetus is stressed as a result of

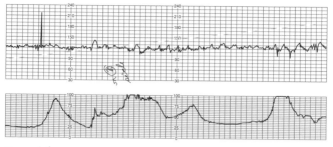

Figure 4-6
Uterine hyperactivity from oxytocin.

diminished placental perfusion and exhibits signs of intolerance to labor, which include decreased FHR variability, persistent late decelerations, and bradycardia.

In addition, hyperstimulation with oxytocics has the potential for uterine rupture. When an oxytocin infusion is discontinued, uterine relaxation usually occurs within 10 minutes, with return of normal baseline FHR and variability. When oxytocin is given by poorly controlled methods, such as the buccal or intramuscular route, there is an added risk because the rate of absorption and any adverse fetal effects are prolonged. The use of the oral or intramuscular route is no longer standard practice because of the potential for adverse consequences. Because hyperstimulation can occur with the use of prostaglandin cervical ripening agents such as dinoprostone and misoprostol, each institution should have policies and procedures outlining the appropriate measures to follow when hyperstimulation occurs with these drugs.

Uterine contractions are known to decrease the rate of blood flow through the intervillous space, and therefore it is important to attentively monitor uterine activity in addition to the FHR. Most fetuses are well able to tolerate this transient type of stress; however, in pregnancies in which the margin of fetal reserve is low, this phenomenon can cause commensurate decreases in FHR (described as late decelerations). The primary care provider should be notified promptly when there is evidence of uterine tachysystole. Notification is especially important when there is uterine hyperstimulation with signs of fetal intolerance to labor that are unresponsive to nursing interventions.

Intervention

1. Discontinue oxytocin if infusing. (Exercise caution in flushing the oxytocin out of the line to ensure that a bolus is not delivered to the woman.)
2. Increase the rate of maintenance intravenous infusion.
3. Change maternal position (lateral preferred).
4. Consider the administration of oxygen, 8 to 10 L/min by face-mask.
5. Notify the primary care provider of the FHR and the uterine activity pattern and the response to interventions already performed.
6. The provider may consider the use of tocolytics such as terbutaline or magnesium sulfate if there is an excessive increase in uterine activity, such as tachysystole or hypertonus, and evidence of a nonreassuring FHR pattern.

Fetal recovery from uterine hyperstimulation is preferred in utero, because once the placental circulation is restored, carbon dioxide from respiratory acidosis, as well as the acidic products of anaerobic metabolism, can be eliminated. Recovery is hampered if delivery occurs prior to the elimination of the anaerobic products.

Inhibition of uterine activity

It is important to decrease uterine activity when premature labor or nonreassuring FHR patterns occur. Drugs such as isoxsuprine, epinephrine, and isoproterenol have been used in the past to reduce uterine activity, but they are not without drawbacks (e.g., their beta-stimulant effects cause vasodilation and secondary hypotension). Because of these extrauterine effects, beta-mimetic agents are now used. Magnesium sulfate is frequently considered the first choice in tocolytic therapy, and terbutaline is routinely used because it has maximal tocolytic effect. The drugs in the following list are known to inhibit uterine activity.

- Beta-sympathomimetics (e.g., terbutaline)
- Magnesium sulfate
- Calcium-channel blockers (e.g., nifedipine)
- Prostaglandin inhibitors (e.g., indomethacin)
- Diazoxide
- Halothane
- Progesterone

Acute tocolysis may be indicated in specific urgent situations. This is discussed in Chapter 6, Assessment and Management of Fetal Status.

References

American College of Obstetricians and Gynecologists (ACOG): Dystocia and augmentation of labor, *Practice Bulletin* no. 49, Washington, DC, December, 2003, The College.

American College of Obstetricians and Gynecologists: Induction of labor, *Practice Bull* no. 10, November, 1999a, The College.

American College of Obstetricians and Gynecologists: Induction of labor with misoprostol. *Committee Opinion* no. 28, Washington, DC, November, 1999b, The College.

Association of Women's Health, Obstetric, and Neonatal Nurses (AWHONN): *Fetal heart monitoring: Principles and practices,* ed 3, Dubuque, Iowa, 2003, Kendall/Hunt.

Caldeyro-Barcia R, Poseiro JJ: Physiology of uterine contractions, *Clin Obstet Gynecol* 3:386-408, 1960.

Dickason EJ, Silverman BL, Kaplan JA: *Maternal–infant nursing care,* ed 3, St Louis, 1998, Mosby.

Freeman RK, Garite TJ, Nageotte MP: *Fetal heart rate monitoring,* Baltimore, 2003, Williams & Wilkins.

Lowdermilk DL, Perry SE: *Maternity & women's health care,* ed 8, St Louis, 2004, Mosby.

McKenzie IZ: Labor induction including pregnancy termination for fetal anomaly. In James DK, Steer PJ, Weiner CP, Gonick B, editors: *High risk pregnancy: Management options,* Philadelphia, 1999, Saunders.

Parer J: *Handbook of fetal heart rate monitoring,* Philadelphia, 1997, Saunders.

Pattern Recognition and Interpretation

Since the advent and widespread use of electronic fetal monitoring, various descriptive terms have been used to describe fetal heart rate (FHR) patterns. The definitions of these terms have not always been globally consistent among practitioners and institutions, resulting in variation in interpretation of FHR tracings. In addition, this lack of standardization and consistency in definitions and nomenclature for FHR patterns has been an impediment to progress in the investigation and evaluation of FHR monitoring.

The National Institute of Child Health and Human Development (NICHD) brought together clinicians, experts in electronic fetal monitoring, from the United States, Canada, and the United Kingdom (NICHD, 1997). Their purpose was to standardize a clear set of definitions that could be quantitated, thus providing a foundation for electronic fetal monitoring terminology used in practice and research. Through the standardized definitions, the predictive value of monitoring can be assessed more meaningfully in appropriately designed observational studies and clinical trials. The hope is that the resulting research-based investigative interpretation will lead to a more evidence-based clinical management of nonreassuring fetal status.

The NICHD definitions were developed primarily for visual FHR interpretation, but they are intended to apply also to computerized interpretation. Definitions apply to FHR patterns produced from either a direct fetal spiral electrode detecting the fetal electrocardiogram (FECG) or an external Doppler ultrasound device detecting the fetal heart events using the autocorrelation technique. Although the prime emphasis of the definitions is on intrapartum patterns, they are also applicable to antepartum observations. The NICHD definitions are used as a basis for the content in this chapter.

Baseline Fetal Heart Rate

Definition

Baseline FHR is the average (mean) FHR rounded to increments of five beats per minute (bpm) during a 10-minute segment of a tracing. The baseline FHR excludes the following:

- Periods of marked FHR variability
- Periodic and episodic changes
- Segments of baseline that differ by more than 25 bpm

In any 10-minute segment, the minimum baseline duration must be at least 2 minutes; otherwise, the baseline is considered to be indeterminate. In this case, the baseline FHR may need to be determined from a previous 10-minute segment. The normal range of FHR at term is 110 to 160 bpm (NICHD, 1997).

Baseline rate is evaluated, assessed, and documented as a range and not as one number (unless variability is absent). Baseline represents the normal fluctuations and irregularities of the fetal heartbeats as they vary from one to the next (Martin, 2002).

Description

Baseline FHR is set by the atrial pacemaker and balanced by an interplay between the sympathetic (cardioaccelerator) and parasympathetic (decelerator) branches of the autonomic nervous system. As a result of the immaturity of the central nervous system and the sympathetic dominance, the premature fetus at approximately 20 weeks of gestation may exhibit a baseline heart rate of 150 to 170 bpm. In the healthy full-term infant, the rate is usually between 110 and 160 bpm (RCOG, 2001). This is the result of the balanced regulatory interaction between parasympathetic and sympathetic nervous systems. A fetus over the age of 40 weeks of gestation may have a rate between 110 and 120 bpm. This rate indicates a slightly greater influence of parasympathetic control.

Assessment of the baseline FHR can be facilitated during periods when there is no stress or stimulation to the fetus. The following guidelines may be used for choosing such a period, especially when it is difficult to assess the baseline FHR (Figure 5-1):

- When the woman is not in labor
- When the fetus is not moving
- Between uterine contractions
- When there is no stimulation to the fetus (as would occur with vaginal examinations and placement of an internal monitoring device)

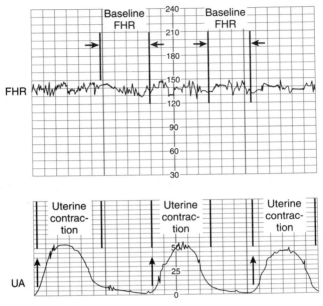

Figure 5-1
Baseline FHR is usually easier to assess between uterine contractions.

■ During the interval between periodic changes (decelerations or accelerations)

Variability

Definition

Baseline FHR variability is defined as fluctuations in the baseline FHR of two cycles per minute or greater. These fluctuations are irregular in amplitude and frequency and are visually quantitated as the amplitude (from peak to trough) in beats per minute, as described in the following chart (NICHD, 1997) (Figure 5-2).

Descriptive Term	Amplitude Range
Absent	Undetectable
Minimal	Just detectable to ≤5 bpm
Moderate (average)	6 to 25 bpm
Marked	>25 bpm

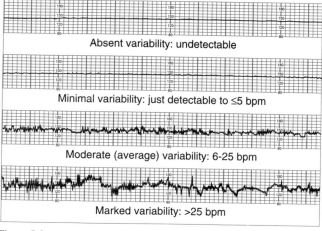

Figure 5-2
Classification of variability.

Description

Variability of the FHR can be described as the normal irregularity of cardiac rhythm, resulting from a continuous balancing interaction of the sympathetic (cardioacceleration) and parasympathetic (cardiodeceleration) branches of the autonomic nervous system. These two branches interact, modulating the FHR. Changes in variability are predominately transmitted through the parasympathetic nervous system. Variability is believed to result from multiple sporadic impulses from the cerebral cortex and the lower centers of the medulla (Martin, 2002). Impulses from these areas then travel down the vagus nerve to the heart.

Moderate or average variability of the FHR is demonstrated by fluctuations of the baseline, which reflect an intact neurological pathway, optimal fetal oxygenation, and an adequate fetal oxygen reserve in the tissue. In addition, intrapartum baseline variability indirectly indicates fetal tolerance of labor.

Short-term and long-term variability

In the NICHD definitions, no distinction is made between short-term variability (STV) and long-term variability (LTV). In actual practice, STV and LTV are viewed together and determined visually as a unit. In addition, the definition of variability excludes the sinusoidal pattern discussed later in this chapter, because this pattern has a smooth sine wave of regular frequency and amplitude. Variability is a characteristic of baseline FHR and does not include either accelerations or decelerations.

Although the definition of variability is objective and clear for visual interpretation, the characteristics of STV and LTV can be distinguished. STV is the beat-to-beat change in FHR from one heartbeat to the next. STV is often described as "present" or "absent." STV reflects the internal difference between successive R peaks of the FECG signal (Figure 5-3). It is a reflection of the normal irregularity in the interval between consecutive heartbeats (cardiac rhythm) and is controlled by the parasympathetic nervous system. Direct ECG (by spiral electrode) is the only method that can accurately measure STV (ACOG, 1995). STV is the sensitive indicator of fetal oxygenation and oxygen reserve in the tissue. The presence of STV is reassuring in that it indicates that the fetus appropriately responds to nerve impulses and has an intact autonomic nervous system.

Long-term variability, on the other hand, is influenced by the sympathetic nervous system. It appears as rhythmic fluctuations in FHR, excluding accelerations, decelerations, and any aberrant marks and artifacts (Table 5-1). Interpretation of LTV is made

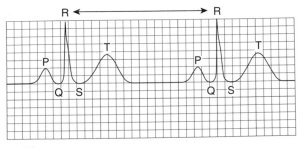

Figure 5-3
The fetal spiral electrode obtains the direct fetal electrocardiogram (DECG), measuring the interval between consecutive fetal R waves. A cardiotachometer converts the interval between R waves to a rate in beats per minute, which is printed on the monitor tracing. This illustration demonstrates the time interval between R waves. However, in the healthy fetus the intervals should vary, showing variability in the FHR from one beat to the next.

by visual examination of the rise and fall (amplitude) and the frequency of changes in the FHR within the baseline range. The frequency of fluctuations can be determined by counting the number of complete cycles per minute, the number of turning points, or the number of times the FHR crosses over an imaginary line, determined as the average or median of the baseline FHR range, within 1 minute (AWHONN, 2003). The presence of LTV gives an indication of fetal oxygenation and the physiological ability to compensate for stress. The absence of LTV may be a marker for fetal hypoxemia and indicates the need for implementation of interventions that will attempt to improve fetal oxygenation.

Generally, STV and LTV tend to increase and decrease together. This is because of the interplay between the parasympathetic and sympathetic nervous systems and their response to external and internal factors. There are also certain instances when STV and LTV exhibit changes independently from each other (Figure 5-4). For example, when a fetus is sleeping, STV may be present and LTV decreased. There are also fetal conditions, such as fetal anemia, that result in FHR patterns in which LTV is present but STV is absent. When evaluating STV and LTV, and when determining whether variability is reassuring or nonreassuring, other factors should be considered, including gestational age (Figure 5-5), drugs, stage of labor, anesthesia, obstetrical history,

Table 5-1   Fetal heart rate (FHR) variability

Type of Variability	Short-Term	Long-Term
Description	A change in FHR from one beat to the next; beat-to-beat variability; normal irregularity of the fetal heart	Rhythmical and cyclical fluctuations in FHR of ≥2 cycles per minute
Appearance		
Signal Source	Spiral electrode	Spiral electrode and ultrasound transducer

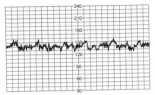

Both short- and
long-term variability

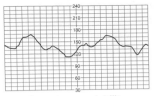

Long-term variability,
absence of short-term variability

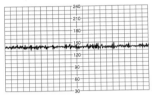

Short-term variability,
absence of long-term variability

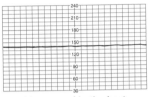

Absence of both short-
and long-term variability

Figure 5-4
Variations in short- and long-term variability.

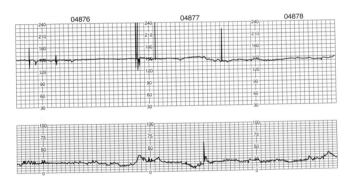

Figure 5-5
Baseline variability is minimal in the first half of the tracing
and then demonstrates a small increase. This fetus was
3 weeks past the due date and later delivered spontaneously
with a meconium-stained placenta, birth weight of 4067 g,
and Apgar scores of 4 at 1 minute and 7 at 5 minutes of age.

prenatal course, fetal condition, and the presence of fetal anomalies. Information about these factors helps to determine the potential need for interventions.

Etiology

The following chart lists causes of increased and decreased variability with their clinical significance and potential interventions.

Cause of Variability	Clinical Significance/Intervention
Marked variability	
1. Mild hypoxemia An early compensatory mechanism produces an increase in STV.	1. The significance of marked (e.g., *saltatory*) variability is not known. It is thought that parasympathetic stimulation does not predominate over sympathetic stimulation, and the result is larger fluctuations in rate, reflecting the interplay between factors that increase heart rate. Marked variability caused by mild hypoxemia does not generally persist and is not associated with progressing hypoxemia (Parer, 1997).
2. Fetal stimulation External uterine palpation, uterine contractions, fetal activity, application of internal monitoring devices, vaginal examination, acoustic stimulation, and maternal activity stimulate the fetal autonomic nervous system, resulting in increased variability.	2. Marked variability caused by fetal stimulation may represent a shifting of Po_2 and Pco_2 mediated by baroreceptors and chemoreceptors. There is no significant change in oxygen unless repetitive decelerations accompany the marked variability. Assess for cause of repetitive late decelerations and perform conventional therapies to treat (e.g., repositioning, hydration, oxygen).
3. Drugs *Stimulants* Initial response to cocaine, crack, and methamphetamines is CNS excitability.	3. Baseline variability should be evaluated before the administration of any drugs. Intervention is not required unless a nonreassuring FHR pattern develops.

Cause of Variability	Clinical Significance/Intervention

Sympathomimetics
  Sympathetic response to terbutaline, and asthma medications may cause maternal and fetal tachycardia in addition to increased variability.

Decreased variability

1. Hypoxemia and acidemia Uteroplacental insufficiency from several causes (uterine hyperstimulation, maternal supine hypotension, amnionitis).

2. Drugs
  Analgesics, narcotics, tranquilizers, barbiturates, and general anesthetics depress CNS mechanisms responsible for cardiac control. Parasympatholytics such as atropine block the transmission of impulses to the sinoatrial (SA) node.

1. Decreasing variability can be an indication of a *nonreassuring fetal status.* Absence of variability exhibited by a smooth or flat baseline is a nonreassuring sign. A flat or smooth baseline associated with late decelerations of *any* magnitude is a sign of hypoxemia and acidemia that is related to CNS depression. Efforts to improve and optimize fetal oxygenation and uteroplacental blood flow through maternal positioning, hydration, correction of maternal hypotension, maternal oxygenation, and elimination of uterine hyperactivity are indicated. Application of a spiral electrode should be considered if the pattern is observed by external monitoring and the tracing is of poor quality.

2. Variability should be evaluated before administration of analgesics and narcotics. Administration time and effect of medications given must be documented. Decreased variability related to drugs usually returns to previous amount of variability as the drug is excreted. If a CNS-depressant drug has been given near the time of delivery,

Cause of Variability	Clinical Significance/Intervention
	naloxone (Narcan) may be administered to the neonate after delivery. Baseline variability should be evaluated before administration of analgesic narcotics and other drugs. Administration time and effect of drugs must be documented. Variability that is decreased as a result of fetal sleep cycles usually resumes in 20 to 40 min.
3. Fetal sleep cycles Fetal sleep cycles produce decreased LTV but do not usually affect STV.	3. Variability that is decreased as a result of fetal sleep usually resumes in 20 to 40 min. In some fetuses, the cycle may last as long as 90 min.
4. Congenital anomalies Central nervous system (e.g., anencephaly) or cardiac anomalies can result in decreased variability.	4. Interventions cannot reverse congenital anomalies.
5. Fetal cardiac arrhythmias Suppression of cardiac control mechanisms may be the result of paroxysmal atrial tachycardia, complete heart block, nodal rhythm, or an aberrant pacemaker.	5. Some cardiac drugs may be given to the woman in an attempt to convert certain fetal dysrhythmias.
6. Extreme prematurity (<24 weeks of gestation) Heartbeat is controlled by immature neurological mechanisms resulting in even intervals from one heartbeat to the next.	6. Heartbeat is normal for gestational age; no intervention is necessary.

Clinical Significance

In summary, variability is considered to be the *most important FHR characteristic.* It reflects neurological modulation of the FHR. Moderate variability indicates that the fetus has an intact autonomic nervous system, the capability to centralize available oxygen, and the ability to compensate for periods of physiologic stress. This is reassuring sign.

If the intervals between successive heartbeats were exactly the same, as in the regular rhythm of a ticking clock or a metronome, the baseline would be flat, indicating central nervous system depression associated with hypoxemia or a previous insult with some CNS impairment. Therefore absence of variability of the FHR is demonstrated by a smooth or flat baseline. Generally, short- and long-term variability increase and decrease together. The absence of long-term variability may be a marker for fetal hypoxemia, and it indicates the need for implementation of interventions that will attempt to improve fetal oxygenation. Unless the absence of variability can be attributed to a temporary cause such as a fetal sleep state, or a reversible cause such as a prescribed CNS depressant, it is considered nonreassuring.

Intervention
Increased baseline variability

Observe the FHR tracing carefully for any sign of nonreassuring fetal status, including periodic changes and increases or decreases in baseline FHR. Consider using an internal spiral electrode if the pattern is observed during external monitoring, especially if there is a concern of change in fetal condition and a decreased tolerance of labor.

Decreased baseline variability

Intervention depends on the cause. Intervention is not warranted if decreased variability is associated with fetal sleep cycles or if it is temporarily associated with prescribed CNS depressants. Application of a spiral electrode should be considered if the pattern is observed during external monitoring and the quality of the tracing is not consistently interpretable. If a CNS-depressant drug has been given near the time of delivery, naloxone may be administered to the neonate after delivery. If hypoxemia is suspected, turning the woman on her side and administering oxygen may improve oxygen saturation. In addition, hydration and elimination of uterine hyperstimulation may enhance fetal oxygenation and improve uteroplacental blood flow. Fetal pulse oximetry may be considered if there is persistent decreased variability ≤5 bpm for ≥60 minutes that is otherwise unexplained by the clinical situation (e.g., narcotic administration), and if *not* accompanied by persistent late or variable decelerations.

Tachycardia

Definition

Fetal tachycardia is defined as a baseline heart rate of 160 bpm or greater for a duration of 10 minutes or more (NICHD, 1997; Parer, 1997; Freeman et al, 2003).

Description

Tachycardia is the result of an increase in sympathetic tone and a decrease in parasympathetic tone and is sometimes associated with a decrease in or loss of FHR variability (Freeman et al, 2003). Fetal tachycardia usually occurs secondary to maternal fever, beta-sympathomimetic drugs, amnionitis, congenital infection, or hyperthyroidism. A fetus that is less than 32 weeks of gestation may have a normal FHR around 160 bpm. As gestational age increases, baseline FHR gradually decreases. Tachycardia may be a sign of early fetal hypoxemia when associated with periodic changes and decreasing baseline variability. Therefore it is important to assess the FHR for trends, including an increase in baseline rate, a decrease in variability, periodic changes, and the duration of the patterns observed (Figures 5-6 and 5-7).

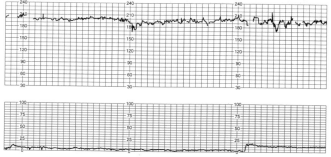

Figure 5-6
Fetal tachycardia with moderate variability.

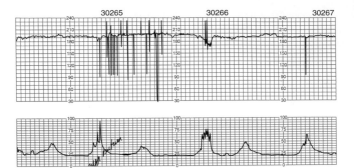

Figure 5-7
Fetal tachycardia, with a mild variable deceleration in panel 30266. Note the wide excursion of vertical lines due to artifact. The baseline rate is not obliterated and can be assessed.

Etiology

Cause of Tachycardia	Mechanism
1. Fetal hypoxemia	1. The fetus attempts to compensate for reduced blood flow by an increase of sympathetic stimulation or a release of epinephrine from adrenal medulla, or both. An increase in cardiac output can be accomplished only by increasing the heart rate.
2. Maternal fever	2. Fever accelerates metabolism of fetal myocardium; it increases sympathetic cardioacceleration activity up to 2 hours before the woman is febrile.
3. Drugs Atropine, hydroxyzine (Vistaril, Atarax), terbutaline, ketamine, phenothiazines (antiemetics, tranquilizers, antipsychotics, antihistamines),	3. Certain drugs have a cardioaccelerator effect on the fetus. Parasympatholytics block the parasympathetic pathway of the autonomic nervous system.

Cause of Tachycardia	Mechanism
dopamine, bronchodilators (e.g., Albuterol), epinephrine, pseudoephedrine decongestants, appetite suppressants, stimulants (e.g., caffeine), illicit drugs such as cocaine and methamphetamines	Beta-sympathomimetics have a cardiac stimulant effect. Other drugs produce an epinephrine/norepinephrine response and cause increases in maternal and fetal heart rates.
4. Amnionitis	4. An increased heart rate can be the first sign of a developing intrauterine infection (as with prolonged rupture of membranes).
5. Maternal hyperthyroidism	5. Long-acting thyroid-stimulating hormones (LATS) probably cross the placenta and increase FHR.
6. Fetal anemia	6. The FHR increases in an effort to increase cardiac output and tissue perfusion.
7. Fetal heart failure	7. The fetal heart attempts to compensate for failure by concurrently increasing rate and cardiac output; this can occur as a result of tachyarrhythmia.
8. Fetal cardiac arrhythmias*	8. Tachyarrhythmias and variations of normal sinus rhythm may occur; a congenital cardiac anomaly may be present; an FHR in excess of 240 bpm cannot be followed by monitor because this exceeds the FHR range parameters (and the rate may be halved because of limitations of the monitor).

*Fetal cardiac arrhythmias (p. 118) may be confused with electrical noise or maternal ECG artifact on the fetal monitor because they are characterized by large vertical excursions on the FHR tracing. They can, however, be diagnosed through the use of a spiral electrode, with M-mode and real-time ultrasound, and by turning off the logic switch on the fetal monitor.

Clinical Significance

Most fetal tachycardias do not reflect a hypoxemic fetus, especially in a term gestation with an identifiable cause such as maternal fever or drugs. However, when seen in a preterm fetus or a term gestation *without* an identifiable cause, further assessment is critical (Freeman et al, 2003).

Three types of fetal tachycardia are sinus tachycardia, atrial flutter/fibrillation, and supraventricular tachycardia. Sinus tachycardia with a rate above 160 bpm may be the result of a drug effect or a response to maternal infection such as amnionitis. It is not necessarily a sign of fetal hypoxemia unless it is associated with repetitive late decelerations and/or a lack of variability. Atrial flutter/fibrillation, with an atrial rate between 400 and 500 bpm, is rarely diagnosed in the antepartum period and is associated with a high mortality rate.

Supraventricular tachycardia (SVT), with a heart rate in excess of 220 bpm, is the most frequently occurring form of fetal tachyarrhythmia. Short periods of SVT are of no clinical significance. However, longer periods of SVT have been associated with fetal cardiac failure, nonimmune hydrops fetalis, ascites, hydramnios, and fetal death.

Tachycardia can be a nonreassuring sign when associated with late decelerations or absence of variability. In terms of immediate neonatal outcome, persistent tachycardia with moderate (average) baseline variability or in the absence of periodic changes (e.g., decelerations) does not appear to adversely compromise the fetus and is rarely associated with fetal asphyxia. This is particularly true when the tachycardia is associated with maternal fever.

Intervention

Intervention for tachycardia depends on the etiological factors. Maternal fever can be reduced with antipyretics and hydration. If maternal oxygenation is an issue, 100% oxygen at 8 to 10 L/min via facemask may improve or optimize fetal oxygenation by supersaturating the maternal plasma oxygen levels. If the FHR is greater than 160 bpm with minimal variability for more than 60 minutes and is not otherwise explained by the clinical situation (e.g., narcotic administration), fetal pulse oximetry may provide additional clinical data.

When the diagnosis of supraventricular tachycardia is made, in utero therapy of the premature fetus or delivery of the mature fetus must be initiated. In utero treatment can consist of maternal administration of a single drug or combinations of digoxin, calcium-channel blockers (nifedipine), beta-blockers (propranolol [Inderal]), and antiarrhythmic agents such as procainamide and quinidine, which cross the placental barrier and treat the fetus.

Bradycardia

Definition

Fetal bradycardia is defined as a baseline heart rate of 110 bpm or less for a duration of 10 minutes or more (NICHD, 1997; Parer, 1997).

Description

Bradycardia is frequently the response of the fetus to hypoxemia; however, nonacidemic causes of bradycardia include heart block and congenital cardiac anomalies. When bradycardia is detected at the initiation of monitoring, it is difficult to distinguish it from a prolonged deceleration. When associated with periodic changes and decreasing baseline variability, bradycardia is generally a late sign of fetal hypoxemia indicative of progressive acidemia. Therefore it is important to assess the FHR for a decrease in baseline rate, a decrease in variability, periodic changes, and the duration of the patterns observed (Figures 5-8 and 5-9).

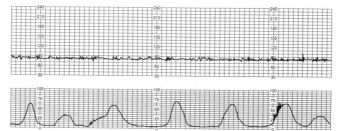

Figure 5-8
Fetal bradycardia.

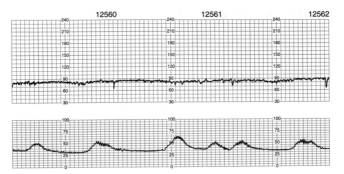

Figure 5-9
Fetal bradycardia.

Etiology

Cause of Bradycardia	Mechanism
1. Late (profound) fetal hypoxemia	1. Myocardial activity becomes depressed and lowers the heart rate.
2. Beta-adrenergic blocking drugs (e.g., propranolol)	2. Epinephrine receptor sites in the myocardium are blocked by these drugs, permitting unopposed vagal tone and a decreased heart rate.
3. Anesthetics (epidural, spinal, and pudendal)	3. Bradycardia may develop indirectly because of a reflex mechanism or because of maternal hypotension produced by maternal supine position, insufficient preanesthesia hydration, or the sympathetic blockade response to the anesthetic agent.
4. Maternal hypotension	4. Maternal supine position causes uterine compression of the vena cava, which results in hypotension syndrome (a decrease in maternal cardiac output and blood pressure, which decreases uteroplacental blood flow, resulting in a subsequent decrease in FHR).

Cause of Bradycardia	Mechanism
5. Prolonged umbilical cord compression	5. Cord compression triggers sensitization of fetal baroceptors, resulting in vagal stimulation and a decreased heart rate.
6. Hypothermia	6. Maternal (and therefore fetal) hypothermia reduces myocardial metabolism, decreases oxygen requirements, and decreases heart rate.
7. Maternal systemic lupus erythematosus	7. Complete atrioventricular dissociation associated with connective tissue disease produces persistent bradycardia.
8. Cytomegalovirus (CMV)	8. Structural cardiac defects may occur with CMV infection, resulting in congenital heart block expressed as fetal bradycardia.
9. Prolonged maternal hypoglycemia	9. Maternal and subsequently fetal hypoglycemia can potentiate hypoxemia with a depression of myocardial activity and a decreased heart rate.
10. Fetal cardiac arrhythmias	10. FHR can be low (70 to 90 bpm) with bradyarrhythmias (complete heart block).
11. Congenital heart block	11. Congenital heart block of the first, second, or third degree can result in bradycardia. First-degree block does not require treatment of the fetus. In second-degree block, not all the impulses from the sinoatrial node in the atria are conducted to the ventricles. A Mobitz type I block is evidenced by a progressive lengthening of the PR interval and is rarely of any significance. A Mobitz type II block occurs infrequently but is more serious and often a precursor to third-degree, or complete, heart block. Complete heart block is most often associated with congenital heart disease.

Clinical Significance

Bradycardia resulting from hypoxemia is a nonreassuring sign when associated with loss of variability and late decelerations. Substantial bradycardia with absent baseline variability, especially when prolonged and uncorrectable, is predictive of current or impending fetal acidemia of such severity that the fetus is at risk of neurological and other fetal damage or death (NICHD, 1997). Bradycardia in the 90- to 110-bpm range with moderate (average) FHR variability and absence of late decelerations is generally reassuring and may be a normal variant for the fetus (Garite, 2002; Freeman et al, 2003). Intervention is also not warranted in a fetus with heart block diagnosed in the antepartum period.

Although paracervical blocks are rarely performed, the resultant bradycardia is usually transitory, with recovery occurring in utero. The 5-minute Apgar score is usually above 7 if the FHR pattern was reassuring before the onset of the bradycardia and if delivery does not occur during the paracervical block bradycardia. Poor fetal outcome has occurred with delivery during the resulting bradycardia caused by fetal hypoxemia and acidemia. Neonatal resuscitation and stabilization is indicated until the paracervical pharmacological agent has been metabolized.

Intervention

Intervention for bradycardia depends on the etiological factors. Clinical judgment and resulting intervention are based on a variety of factors, including stage of labor, presentation and station of fetus, and indications of fetal status. Maternal positioning (lateral), hydration, correction of maternal hypotension, maternal oxygenation at 10 L/min at 100% by facemask, and elimination of uterine activity and/or hyperstimulation are indicated to optimize and improve fetal oxygenation. Infants delivered with congenital heart block may require a pacemaker.

Unusual Patterns
Sinusoidal Pattern

A sinusoidal FHR pattern (Figures 5-10 and 5-11) is a *sine* wave characterized by an *undulating* baseline and the following features:

- Regular oscillations with an amplitude range of 5 to 15 bpm
- Frequency of undulations of two to five cycles per minute of long-term variability

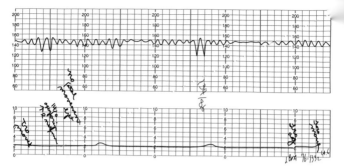

Figure 5-10

Sinusoidal pattern. Note the characteristic regularity and smoothness.

(Courtesy Roger K. Freeman, Long Beach, Calif.)

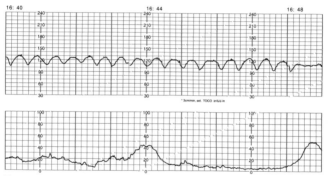

Figure 5-11

Sinusoidal fetal heart rate. Note the rhythmic undulating pattern.

- Minimal to absent short-term variability
- Rhythmic oscillation of a sine wave above and below a baseline
- Absence of FHR accelerations, whether spontaneous, stimulated, or in response to fetal movement
- Extreme regularity and smoothness

This pattern has been known to occur in the presence of fetal hypoxemia, often as a result of Rh isoimmunization, fetal anemia, and chronic fetal bleeds. In these cases, it has been associated with an increase in fetal morbidity and mortality, and survival may depend on extrauterine support in a neonatal intensive care unit.

A *pseudosinusoidal* pattern has also been reported after the administration of narcotics, opioid analgesics (such as meperidine),

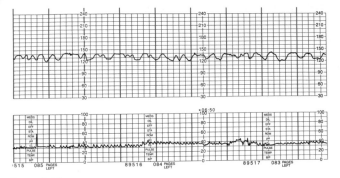

Figure 5-12
Pseudosinusoidal pattern. This pattern is neither regular nor smooth. Although narcotics may cause this type of pattern, they were not the cause in this case. This could have been caused by amnionitis, or by fetal sucking or mouthing motions. This particular pattern was preceded and followed by a period of accelerations.

and butorphanol tartrate (Stadol), in association with amnionitis and with fetal thumb-sucking. The pattern following the administration of narcotics is usually a temporary phenomenon not associated with an adverse fetal outcome. Pseudosinusoidal patterns are characterized by sine waves that are less uniform, and STV is usually present (Figure 5-12). In addition, these patterns are preceded and followed by normal FHR patterns.

Notify the health care provider if this pattern is detected on admission or without other identifiable causes. If there is a persistent, uncorrectable sinusoidal pattern and other signs of fetal compromise are present, expeditious delivery may be indicated. If the pattern is inconsistent and apparently transitory after intravenous narcotics, nonreassuring fetal status is not expected.

Fetal Cardiac Arrhythmias
Definition

Fetal arrhythmias, also called dysrhythmias, are deviations from the normal cardiac rhythm, and they occur in many pregnancies. The recognition of fetal arrhythmias has increased as a result of electronic FHR monitoring. Diagnosis can be made with M-mode and real-time ultrasound, and with color-encoded fetal echocardiography.

Types of Arrhythmias	Characteristics and Clinical Significance

1. Tachyarrhythmias

a. Premature atrial contractions (PACs) and premature ventricular contractions (PVCs)

PACs and PVCs appear as vertical excursions above and below the FHR baseline on the monitor tracing; bigeminy or trigeminy may also be present. PACs occur more frequently than PVCs. These arrhythmias are often diagnosed in the intrapartum period, do not persist in the neonatal period, and rarely require therapy.

b. Sinus tachycardia

FHR >160 bpm secondary to maternal fever, drugs, amnionitis, congenital infection, hyperthyroidism. This is generally a benign pattern, not associated with hypoxemia unless associated with severe variable decelerations or late decelerations.

c. Atrial flutter/fibrillation

Atrial rate may be between 400 and 500 bpm. Fibrillation is rarer in the fetus than flutter. This arrhythmia is rarely diagnosed in the antepartum period and is often associated with a high mortality rate.

d. Supraventricular tachycardia (SVT)

SVT is characterized by FHR ≥220 bpm with absent variability. This is the most frequently occurring form of fetal tachyarrhythmia. Short periods of SVT may occur intermittently and are of no clinical significance. Long periods of SVT are associated with cardiac failure, nonimmune hydrops fetalis, and fetal death.

2. Bradyarrhythmias

First-, second-, and third-degree heart block

FHR <100 bpm with progressive pro-longation of the P-R interval associated with first-, second-, or third-degree (complete) congenital heart block. First-degree heart block does not require treatment of the fetus. In second-degree block, not all the impulses from the sinoatrial node are conducted to the ventricles. There are two forms of second-degree block: Mobitz types I and II. Mobitz type I block is evidenced

Types of Arrhythmias	Characteristics and Clinical Significance
	by a progressive lengthening of the P-R interval and is rarely of any significance. Mobitz type II block is evidenced by a fixed P-R interval, occurs infrequently, and is more serious and often a precursor to third-degree, or complete, heart block. Complete heart block is usually associated with congenital heart disease or autoimmune disease and is characterized by an FHR of between 40 and 60 bpm. Postdelivery intervention is usually successful in the fetus without congenital heart disease. High mortality is associated with nonimmune hydrops from heart failure, and with congenital cardiac malformations.

It is important to distinguish fetal arrhythmias from electrical noise or maternal ECG artifact, because they can be evidenced by similar patterns (Figure 5-13). A diagnosis that adequately discriminates between fetal arrhythmia and noise/artifact can be achieved by spiral electrode, real-time ultrasound, turning off the logic switch, and checking the electronic fetal monitor for malfunction. With arrhythmias, the FHR baseline can usually be seen between the vertical lines on the tracing (Gilbert, Harmon, 2003) (Figure 5-14). Artifact, on the other hand, appears as irregular vertical lines on a tracing that has previously recorded a regular baseline rate and rhythm. In addition, artifact obscures the baseline fetal heart rate (Gilbert, Harmon, 2003).

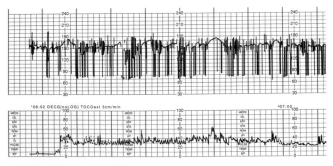

Figure 5-13
Fetal cardiac arrhythmia of premature ventricular contractions.

Isolated extrasystoles, most of which are supraventricular in origin, are of little clinical importance and are the major disturbance of fetal cardiac rhythm. On auscultation, this sounds like a skipped beat, but it is usually either a pause after an extrasystole or an undetectable heartbeat. The majority of fetal cardiac arrhythmias resolve spontaneously in late pregnancy or during the first few days after birth. The treatment of arrhythmias is one of the most specialized disciplines of cardiology and not without significant potential risk of undesired effects. Use of antiarrhythmic drugs must be based on a thorough understanding of the electrophysiology of the arrhythmia, as well as on the electrophysiological and hemodynamic effects of the chemotherapeutic agents. The interactive potential between potent antiarrhythmic agents must be considered as well. The action of these drugs alters the electrophysiological activity of the heart by altering the ion flux at the level of the ion channels within the cell membrane. Drug interactions at the cellular level have the potential for impairing myocardial performance and interfering with metabolism of other drugs, and they could result in a proarrhythmic effect—that is, they may cause rather than ameliorate an arrhythmia.

On occasion, antiarrhythmic therapy is initiated in specialized tertiary centers on an inpatient basis after a risk–benefit analysis and after consultation with the obstetrician, pediatric cardiologist, and informed parents. The fetus is continually monitored before, during, and after administration of the antiarrhythmic agent to the woman. The woman is monitored with a diagnostic 12-lead ECG, a continuous 5-lead ECG, and baseline and ongoing maternal blood studies (Kleinman et al, 1999).

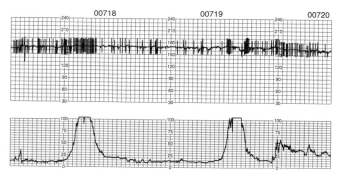

Figure 5-14
Fetal cardiac arrhythmia. Note that the baseline FHR is about 170 bpm.

The following chart is a summary of baseline FHR changes.

Tachycardia	
Definition	Sustained FHR above 160 bpm for >10 min
Etiology	Early hypoxemia, drugs, maternal fever, amnionitis, fetal anemia, fetal heart failure, and/or cardiac dysrhythmias
Clinical significance	Usually benign when associated with maternal fever
	Nonreassuring when associated with a loss of variability, late or severe variable decelerations
Nursing intervention	Depending on etiologic factors, reduce maternal fever with hydration and antipyretics, lateral position change, and oxygen at 10 L/min by facemask.
	For supraventricular tachycardia, in utero treatment can consist of maternal administration of a single drug or a combination of digoxin, calcium-channel blocker (Inderal), and antiarrhythmic agents such as procainamide and quinidine, all of which cross the placenta barrier and treat the fetus.

Bradycardia	Minimal to Absent Variability
Sustained FHR below 110 bpm for >10 min	*Baseline variability:* rhythmic fluctuations in the baseline FHR >2 cycles per minute; irregular in amplitude and frequency
	Short term: changes in FHR from one beat to the next
Late (profound) fetal hypoxemia, drugs, maternal hypotension, prolapsed cord, congenital heart block	*Decreased variability:* prematurity, drugs, hypoxemia, fetal sleep, congenital anomalies, fetal cardiac arrhythmias, CNS depression
Bradycardia of 100 to 110 bpm without periodic deceleration and with average variability is not usually a sign of fetal hypoxemia.	Benign when associated with periodic fetal sleep; return of variability usually occurs when drugs are excreted or metabolized
Nonreassuring when associated with late decelerations or a loss of variability	Nonreassuring when associated with late, severe variable decelerations or a baseline change
Depends on etiological factors. Lateral position change and oxygen at 10 L/min by facemask may be of some value; eliminate uterine tachysystole or hyperstimulation to improve fetal oxygenation and uteroplacental blood flow. Intervention is not warranted in the fetus with heart block diagnosed by ECG in the antepartum period.	Depends on etiological factors. Intervention is not warranted if associated with fetal sleep cycle or temporarily associated with CNS depressants. It is appropriate to provide conventional therapies to improve variability, which include oxygen by facemask, repositioning to a lateral position, providing an increase in circulating volume with intravenous fluids, performing stimulation (between contractions and any periodic changes) in an effort to produce an acceleration, or performing a fetal acoustic stimulation test (FAST) for the same reason. Fetal pulse oximetry may be considered for tachycardia >160 bpm for >60 min with minimal variability that is not otherwise explained (e.g., narcotic administration).

Periodic and Episodic Changes

Periodic changes in fetal heart rate (FHR) are transient accelerations or decelerations from the baseline, after which the FHR returns to baseline. These changes occur in response to uterine contractions (UCs) and may begin as compensatory mechanisms or precursors to hypoxia.

Episodic changes (formerly called nonperiodic changes) are accelerations or decelerations that occur without any specific relationship to uterine activity. They can include spontaneous accelerations and variable decelerations between contractions and prolonged decelerations.

All FHR changes, whether periodic or episodic, should be systematically evaluated within the parameters of the "company they keep" (Chez, 1992). These parameters include FHR baseline and variability before and after the change; presence of combined changes (e.g., lates and variables); change related to uterine activity or resting tone (e.g., hyperactivity and increased resting tone), and general information that is available about maternal and fetal condition. By doing this complete assessment, the clinician remains aware of changes and trends that may suggest a nonreassuring FHR as well as the presence or absence of compensatory mechanisms that give an indication of the level of oxygen reserve in fetal tissue. Timely and appropriate interventions then follow the evaluation of the FHR pattern and a determination of fetal tolerance to labor. By NICHD (1997) criteria, periodic and episodic changes are defined as repetitive if they occur with 50% or more of UCs within 20 minutes.

Accelerations

Definition

Acceleration is defined as a visually apparent, abrupt increase in FHR above the baseline. The onset of the acceleration to its peak is less than 30 seconds. The increase is calculated from the most recently determined portion of the baseline. In the fetus that is older than 32 weeks of gestation, the acme (highest point) is more than 15 bpm above the baseline, and the acceleration lasts more than 15 seconds but less than 2 minutes from the onset of the acceleration to the return to baseline. Before the completion of 32 weeks of gestation, accelerations are defined as having an acme

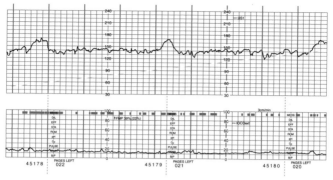

Figure 5-15
Spontaneous (episodic) accelerations.

of more than 10 bpm above the baseline for a duration of more than 10 seconds.

A prolonged acceleration has a duration of 2 minutes or more but less than 10 minutes. An apparent acceleration that lasts 10 minutes or more is a change of FHR baseline (NICHD, 1997).

Description

The majority of accelerations of FHR from the baseline are episodic and *not* associated with uterine contractions. These *episodic* accelerations are most often associated with fetal movement or stimulation and environmental stimuli (Figure 5-15). Episodic (or spontaneous) accelerations of FHR with or without fetal movement are considered reassuring and form the basis for the nonstress test (NST).

When accelerations are associated with uterine contractions, they are considered to be a *periodic* change (Figure 5-16). Repetitive accelerations with UCs are observed less frequently than spontaneous episodic accelerations and may be precursors to variable decelerations.

Characteristics

Characteristics	Episodic/ Spontaneous	Periodic (Associated With Uterine Contractions)
SHAPE	Transitory increase in baseline	Resembles shape of UC; may be biphasic or triphasic

Characteristics	Episodic/ Spontaneous	Periodic (Associated With Uterine Contractions)
ONSET	Can occur at any time; onset to peak, <30 sec	Before or after peak of UC; onset to peak, <30 sec
RECOVERY	Variable; >15 sec to <2 min from onset of acceleration to return to baseline	Return to baseline can occur after or at the same time as uterine pressure returns to its resting tone; ≥15 sec to <2 min from onset of acceleration to return to baseline
ACCELERATION	In the fetus that is >32 weeks of gestation, acceleration is ≥15 bpm above baseline for ≥15 sec; in the fetus that is <32 weeks of gestation, acceleration acme is ≥10 bpm above baseline with a duration of ≥10 sec	Usually ≥15 bpm above baseline for ≥15 sec; if <32 weeks of gestation, acme is ≥10 bpm above baseline with duration of ≥10 sec
BASELINE	Associated with average baseline variability	Sometimes associated with decreasing or smooth baseline variability
OCCURRENCE	Varies; can occur at any time; usually in response to fetal movement or stimulation	Repetitious; tends to occur with each contraction

Etiology

Stimulation of the sympathetic division of the autonomic nervous system can accelerate the fetal heart rate. FHR accelerations can be associated with the following:

- Spontaneous fetal movement
- Vaginal examination
- Abdominal palpation

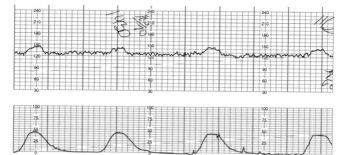

Figure 5-16

Periodic accelerations with uterine contractions.

- Environmental stimuli (e.g., noise)
- Scalp stimulation
- Vibroacoustic stimulation (VAS or FAST)
- Uterine contractions
- Application of the spiral electrode
- Fundal pressure
- Breech presentation
- Occiput posterior presentation
- Insertion of intrauterine pressure catheter (IUPC)

Clinical Significance

Episodic or spontaneous accelerations of FHR in response to fetal movement and fetal stimulation are associated with an intact fetal central nervous system and fetal well-being. Accelerations of FHR in the intrapartum period, whether spontaneous or associated with fetal movement and fetal stimulation, are reassuring. Fetal movement can be identified on the uterine activity (UA) channel as spikes or momentary increases in uterine pressure on the lower section of the monitor tracing. Some electronic fetal monitors have movement sensors that detect and record movement through the ultrasound transducer. Accelerations may be seen in response to stimulation of the fetal head as occurs with vaginal examinations and insertion of a scalp electrode or IUPC.

Repetitive accelerations that are associated with uterine contractions (periodic) may be the earliest indicator of possible partial cord compression (Freeman et al, 2003). This can be secondary to a baroreceptor-induced transient increase in FHR that occurs as a result of fetal hypotension produced when a uterine contraction compresses the umbilical cord. This compensatory mechanism reflects a healthy fetus with an appropriate cardiovascular response.

Intervention

Acceleration of FHR is considered a benign pattern and no intervention is required. If partial cord compression is suspected, maternal repositioning should be done. However, it is recommended that repetitive accelerations in association with uterine contractions be observed in case they evolve into FHR decelerations as labor progresses.

Lambda Pattern

The lambda pattern (Figure 5-17) is common in early labor. It consists of an acceleration followed by a deceleration prior to returning to the baseline. The pattern, which is associated with uterine contractions, does not persist past early labor, and its physiology is unknown. The lambda pattern is not a predictor of the development of a nonreassuring pattern, and it does not require any intervention. It is included here because it does occur at times and should not be confused with a late deceleration or any other nonreassuring pattern (Freeman et al, 2003).

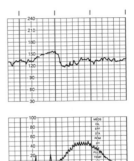

Early Decelerations
Definition

Early deceleration of the fetal heart rate is a periodic change (associated with a uterine contraction). It is a visually apparent *gradual* decrease (defined as the onset of the deceleration to the nadir [lowest point] in 30 seconds or more) and return to the baseline FHR. The decrease is determined from the most recently determined portion of the baseline. It is coincident in timing with the nadir of the deceleration, which occurs at the same time as the peak of the uterine contraction (NICHD, 1997).

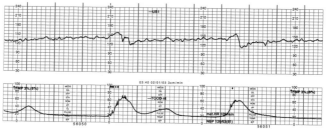

Figure 5-17

Lambda pattern. Note acceleration before deceleration and then return to FHR baseline in association with uterine contractions. Does not require intervention and should not be confused with late decelerations.

Description

Early decelerations are caused by compression of the fetal head, which leads to stimulation of the vagus nerve, resulting in a decrease in the fetal heart rate. Early decelerations begin early in the contracting phase—the onset is before the peak of the uterine contraction—and the recovery occurs at the same time the uterine contraction returns to the baseline. The timing is synchronous with that of the contraction. Generally, this pattern occurs more frequently during the active phase of labor (initially occurring at a point between 4 and 7 cm of dilatation), and it may be present until cervical dilatation is complete at 10 cm. Early decelerations are considered to be benign (ACOG, 1995; Simpson, Creehan, 2002; Freeman et al, 2003).

Physiology

The physiology of early decelerations is described in the accompanying illustration.

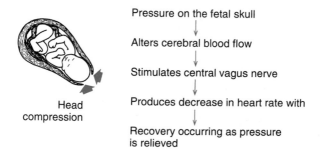

Head compression

Pressure on the fetal skull
↓
Alters cerebral blood flow
↓
Stimulates central vagus nerve
↓
Produces decrease in heart rate with
↓
Recovery occurring as pressure is relieved

Characteristics (Figure 5-18)

SHAPE   Uniform shape; a mirror image of the
                     contraction phase.

ONSET   Early in the contraction phase, before the peak
                     of the contraction. Onset to nadir ≥30 sec;
                     nadir, or low point, of the deceleration
                     occurs at the same time as the peak of the
                     contraction.

RECOVERY   Return to baseline occurs by the end of the
                     contraction as uterine pressure returns to its
                     resting tone.

DECELERATION   Rarely decelerates below 110 bpm, or 30 bpm
                     below baseline; amplitude of deceleration is
                     usually proportional to amplitude of
                     contraction.

BASELINE RATE AND   Usually associated with average baseline rate
   VARIABILITY   and variability.

OCCURRENCE   Repetitious; occurs with each contraction;
                     usually observed between 4 and 7 cm
                     dilatation; observed when there is head
                     compression; occurs most often in
                     primigravidas; often associated with laboring
                     down process, especially with epidural
                     anesthesia.

Etiology

This pattern is caused by direct vagal stimulation of the temporal
baroreceptors from increased pressure and descent of the fetal head
as it passes through the pelvic outlet and vaginal canal. Early
decelerations occur as a result of the following:

- Uterine contractions
- Cephalopelvic disproportion, especially when the pattern occurs
  in early labor
- Persistent occiput posterior

Clinical Significance

Early decelerations, caused by head compression, have no
pathological significance. They do not occur in all labors, but when
they do appear they are repetitive and associated with uterine

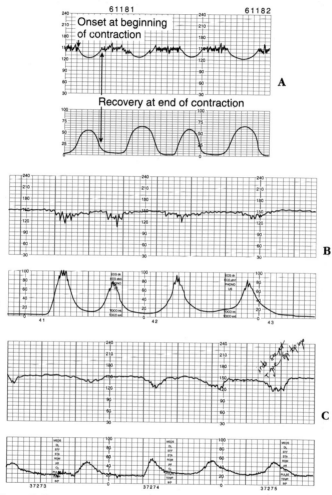

Figure 5-18

A, Early deceleration (illustration, with key points identified).
B and **C,** Early decelerations (actual tracings).

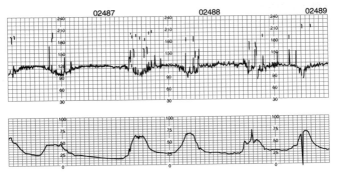

Figure 5-19
Early decelerations occur with each contraction. This is a benign pattern and no intervention is required.

contractions (Figure 5-19). They are not associated with decreasing baseline variability or with changes in baseline FHR.

A *transient deceleration* of FHR may occur with vaginal examinations, placement of the internal scalp electrode or intrauterine pressure catheter, or fundal pressure. Transient decelerations should not be confused with early decelerations, which are a periodic change, repetitive, and associated with uterine contractions.

Intervention

Early decelerations are a benign pattern and no intervention is required. The importance of identifying early decelerations is to be able to distinguish them from late and variable decelerations. The presence of early decelerations should be documented.

Late Decelerations
Definition

Late deceleration of the fetal heart rate is a visually apparent, gradual decrease and return to baseline FHR associated with a uterine contraction. The timing of the onset to nadir is 30 seconds or more. The decrease is determined from the most recently determined portion of the baseline. The deceleration is delayed in time, with the nadir (lowest point) of the deceleration occurring *after* the peak of the contraction (NICHD, 1997).

Description

Late decelerations are those that begin late in the contracting phase. The onset of the deceleration occurs after the onset of the uterine contraction, with the nadir occurring after the peak or acme of the contraction. The recovery of the deceleration occurs after the return of the contraction to the uterine activity baseline. Late decelerations are repetitive periodic changes (associated with uterine contractions) indicative of uteroplacental insufficiency. Therefore they are nonreassuring and require investigation as to cause.

Physiology

The physiology of late decelerations is described in the accompanying illustration.

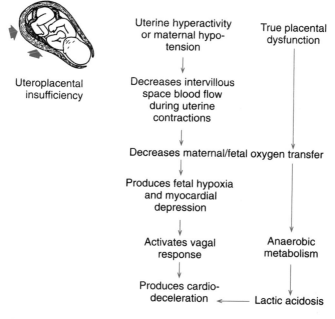

Uteroplacental insufficiency

Uterine hyperactivity or maternal hypotension → Decreases intervillous space blood flow during uterine contractions

True placental dysfunction

Decreases maternal/fetal oxygen transfer

Produces fetal hypoxia and myocardial depression → Activates vagal response → Produces cardiodeceleration

Anaerobic metabolism → Lactic acidosis → Produces cardiodeceleration

Characteristics (Figure 5-20)

SHAPE   Uniform shape; a mirror image of the contraction phase; may be deep or shallow, depending on the degree of hypoxia

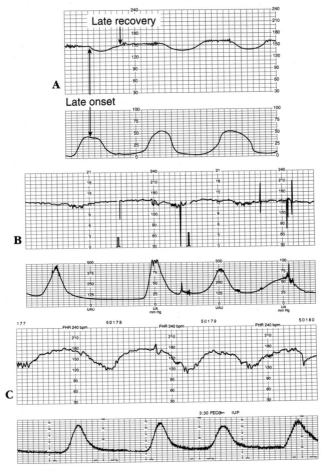

Figure 5-20
A, Late decelerations (illustration, with key points identified).
B and **C,** Late decelerations (actual tracings).

ONSET	Late in the contraction phase; onset to nadir ≥30 sec; nadir, or low point, of the deceleration occurs after the peak of the contraction
RECOVERY	Return to the baseline occurs after the end of the contraction (usually >20 sec after uterine pressure returns to its resting tone)
DECELERATION	Rarely decelerates below 100 bpm; amplitude of deceleration is usually proportional to amplitude of contraction; *persistent, uncorrected* decelerations of *any* magnitude are nonreassuring, and the most depressed fetuses may have only shallow or subtle late decelerations (e.g., 3 to 5 bpm)
BASELINE RATE AND VARIABILITY	Often associated with loss of variability and a rising baseline rate or tachycardia; variability may be increased or decreased during the nadir of the deceleration
OCCURRENCE	Repetitious; occurs with each contraction; can be observed at any time during labor when there is uteroplacental insufficiency (Figure 5-21)

Etiology

Uteroplacental insufficiency can result from the following:

Cause of Uteroplacental Insufficiency	Mechanism
1. Hyperactivity of the uterus from oxytocin augmentation or induction, or from other oxytocic medications	1. Hyperactivity enhances vasoconstriction, reduces cardiac output, and decreases blood flow in the intervillous space.
2. Maternal supine hypotension	2. Compression of the inferior vena cava reduces venous return and maternal cardiac output.
3. Pregnancy-induced hypertension	3. Vasospasm occurring in uterine vessels decreases intervillous space blood flow and produces fetal hypoxemia.
4. Chronic hypertension	4. Hypertensive vascular disease constricts blood vessels and

Cause of Uteroplacental Insufficiency	Mechanism
	reduces intervillous space blood flow, thus producing fetal hypoxemia.
5. Postterm gestation	5. Fetus "outgrows" placenta; insufficient function of the placenta reduces supply of oxygen and nutrients to the fetus.
6. Amnionitis	6. Maternal infection reduces the efficiency of the uteroplacental unit, and related fetal tachycardia increases the metabolic rate, rapidly depleting placental oxygen reserves; amnionitis often causes uterine hyperactivity, which decreases intervillous space blood flow and leads to fetal hypoxemia.
7. Intrauterine growth restriction (IUGR)	7. Poor placental reserve
8. Maternal (poorly controlled or uncontrolled) diabetes	8. Maternal vascular involvement and sclerotic arterial changes reduce uteroplacental perfusion.
9. Placenta previa	9. Placental attachment to the lower uterine segment (covering the internal cervical os) may cause early separation and increase chance of hemorrhage.
10. Abruptio placenta/ maternal shock	10. Premature separation of placenta decreases functioning placental area and related uterine hyperactivity.
11. Regional anesthetics	11. May cause maternal hypotension, reducing blood flow to uteroplacental unit.
12. Maternal cardiac disease	12. Cardiac conditions that affect pumping of blood reduce blood flow to uteroplacental unit; cyanotic conditions reduce oxygen content of blood flowing to placenta.

Cause of Uteroplacental Insufficiency	Mechanism
13. Maternal hematological disorders (e.g., anemia, sickle cell disease)	13. Reduction of red blood cells or hemoglobin decreases the amount of oxygen to fetoplacental unit.
14. Rh isoimmunization	14. Fetal anemia decreases the amount of available oxygen, and the hypoxemic stress occurring with a uterine contraction can precipitate metabolic acidemia.
15. Maternal smoking	15. Contributes to diminished gas exchange through the placenta and can lead to fetal hypoxemia.
16. Other conditions: collagen vascular disease, renal disease, advanced maternal age	16. Placental exchange compromised as a result of sclerotic arterial and venous changes in these conditions.

Clinical Significance

Late decelerations should be considered a nonreassuring sign when they are persistent and uncorrectable. When associated with minimal or absent variability and/or tachycardia, they are a further predictor of fetal acidemia. As myocardial depression increases,

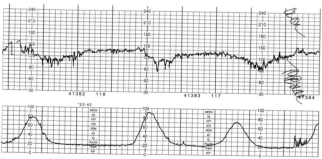

Figure 5-21
Late decelerations.

the depth of the late deceleration decreases, becoming more subtle or shallow. In contrast, a single late deceleration in an otherwise reassuring pattern is not clinically significant. Nonacidemic or "reflex late" decelerations, as described by Parer (1997, p. 163), are late decelerations where moderate (average) variability is retained. This moderate variability is a reflection of an intact fetal CNS.

Persistent and uncorrectable late decelerations reflect repetitive hypoxemic stress and, if associated with minimal or absent variability, are sign of increasing metabolic acidemia.

Intervention for Late Decelerations

Procedure	Rationale
1. Change maternal position to lateral.	1. Decreases pressure on the inferior vena cava, aorta, renal, and uterine arteries; corrects supine hypotension caused by weight of gravid uterus on these vessels; increases maternal cardiac output; increases blood flow to placenta
2. Correct maternal hypotension.	2. Improve uteroplacental blood flow
a. Lower head (unless contraindicated by regional anesthesia).	a. Increases venous return from periphery; promotes maternal cardiac output
b. Provide IV fluid bolus unless contraindicated.	b. Increases maternal circulating volume and cardiac output, improving perfusion of the placenta
c. Administer vasopressors (e.g., ephedrine sulfate) for severe unresponsive hypotension caused by conduction anesthesia.	c. Increases blood pressure by increasing arteriolar constriction and cardiac stimulation
3. Palpate uterus.	3. Determine and assess uterine hyperactivity and/or hypertonus.
4. Discontinue oxytocin if infusing, remove uterotonic agents, consider tocolytics.	4. Decreases uterine activity and increases blood flow to the placenta

Procedure	Rationale
5. Administer oxygen 8-10 L/min by facemask.	5. Hyperoxygenation of maternal blood increases fetal oxygen saturation of hemoglobin, with maximum increase after 8 to 9 min of 100% O_2 to woman (McNamara et al, 1993).
6. Assess maternal vital signs and perform vaginal examination.	6. Determine if maternal condition is contributing to FHR pattern. Clinical status will provide information regarding labor progress.
7. Perform fetal scalp or acoustic stimulation (when FHR is at baseline; *not* during a deceleration).	7. May be useful to elicit an acceleration that would indicate fetal oxygenation status and fetal reserve.
8. Consider internal monitoring.	8. May provide more accurate assessment of fetal and uterine condition.
9. Fetal pulse oximetry may be considered if the pattern is not accompanied by decreased or absent variability.	9. Provides additional data; distinguishes normoxia from hypoxemia in the fetus.
10. Prepare for delivery of fetus if pattern cannot be corrected (particularly if variability is decreasing and acceleration cannot be elicited).	10. Continuation of labor can only further compromise the fetus by increasing hypoxemia and acidemia.

NOTE: Communicate the presence of pattern, interventions, and effects of interventions to care provider and document them. This should occur when it is appropriate on the basis of an assessment of maternal and fetal status. Follow up to ensure that the care provider performs an appropriate and timely assessment of maternal and fetal status, and that this is reflected in the medical record.

Variable Decelerations

Definition

Variable deceleration of the fetal heart rate is defined as a visually apparent *abrupt* decrease in FHR below the baseline. The time from the onset of the deceleration to the beginning of the nadir is less than 30 seconds. The amount of decrease is determined from the most recently determined portion of the baseline. The decrease in FHR below the baseline is 15 or more beats per minute, lasting 15 or more seconds but less than 2 minutes from onset to return to baseline (NICHD, 1997).

Physiology

The physiology of variable decelerations is described in the accompanying illustrations.

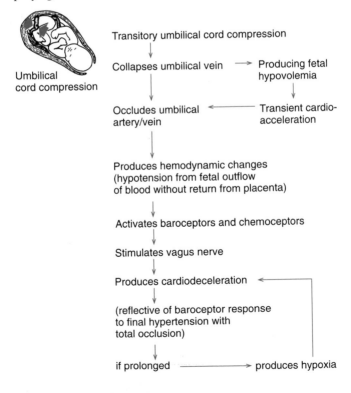

Umbilical cord compression

Transitory umbilical cord compression
↓
Collapses umbilical vein → Producing fetal hypovolemia
↓ ↓
Occludes umbilical ← Transient cardio-acceleration
artery/vein
↓
Produces hemodynamic changes
(hypotension from fetal outflow
of blood without return from placenta)
↓
Activates baroceptors and chemoceptors
↓
Stimulates vagus nerve
↓
Produces cardiodeceleration ←
(reflective of baroceptor response
to final hypertension with
total occlusion)
↓
if prolonged ——————→ produces hypoxia

Description

Variable decelerations are usually episodic changes caused by umbilical cord compression. They can occur with any interruption in umbilical blood flow at any time during labor but are often a periodic change concurrent with uterine contractions. The decelerations vary in the depth of the nadir, and duration is less than 2 minutes. They frequently decelerate below the average FHR range. Variable decelerations are the most frequently observed FHR pattern in labor.

Characteristics (Figures 5-22 to 5-24)

SHAPE	Variable; does not reflect the shape of any associated uterine contraction; characterized by an abrupt drop in heart rate in a V ($\vee$), U ($\cup$), or W (W) shape. All shapes may occur during a labor. There may not be a consistent shape.
ONSET	Variable times in the contraction phase; onset to beginning of nadir, <30 sec; often preceded and followed by transitory acceleration (shouldering)
RECOVERY	Return to baseline occurs rapidly; may have a transitory acceleration before and after UC ($\cup$) (shouldering), or overshoot ($\vee$) (a smooth acceleration after UC); may have a slow gradual return to baseline
DECELERATION	FHR decrease is ≥15 bpm; often decelerates below 100 bpm; lasts ≥15 sec but <2 min. Duration may vary in the same tracing.
BASELINE RATE AND VARIABILITY	May be associated with average baseline rate and variability, or absent variability with significant hypoxia
OCCURRENCE	Observed when there is cord compression; not necessarily repetitive; frequently observed late in labor with descent of fetal head; may be associated with pushing in the second stage of labor

Etiology

Interruption in umbilical blood flow can result from the following:

- Maternal position; cord between fetus and maternal pelvis
- Cord around fetal neck (nuchal cord) or entangled by leg, arm, or other body part
- Short cord
- True knot(s) in cord
- Prolapsed cord
- Oligohydramnios
- After rupture of membrane, when there is a decrease in the amount of protective amniotic fluid cushion

Clinical Significance

Variable decelerations indicate umbilical cord compression. They are the most common deceleration pattern seen in labor and are usually transient and correctable phenomena. They vary in duration, depth (nadir), and timing relative to uterine contractions and any other type of interruption in umbilical blood flow. When variable decelerations are associated with uterine contractions, their onset, depth, and duration commonly vary with successive uterine contractions (NICHD, 1997).

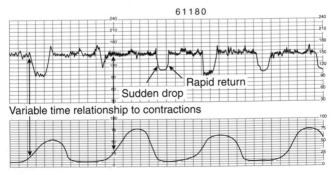

Figure 5-22
Mild variable decelerations (illustration, with key points identified).

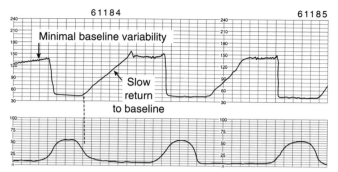

Figure 5-23
Severe variable decelerations (illustration, with key points identified).

Shouldering and overshoot

Shouldering or overshoot may occur with variable decelerations (Figure 5-25). *Shouldering* is a transient preacceleratory and postacceleratory phase of the FHR, generally lasting less than 20 seconds, at the beginning and end of the deceleration. These increases in FHR above the baseline, before and after the variable deceleration has reached its nadir, appear to "shoulder" the deceleration. This is considered to be a normal ("typical") physio-logical compensatory mechanism, usually seen with uterine contractions, and it is reassuring.

Overshoot is a transitory acceleration of the FHR, with a smooth appearance, that occurs at the end of a variable decelera-tion. After the variable deceleration has reached its nadir, the FHR increases and temporarily "overshoots" and then returns to the baseline rate. Overshoots generally follow moderate and severe variable decelerations, have absent variability, and usually last more than 60 seconds.

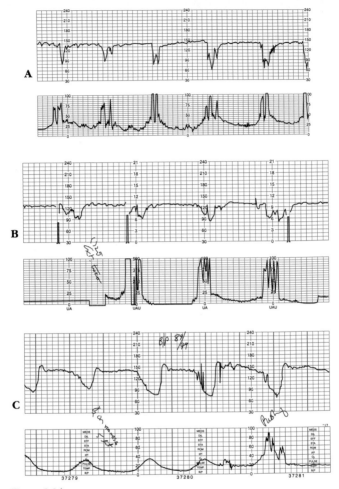

Figure 5-24
Variable decelerations. Note the progression in severity from panel **A** to panel **E**, with overshoots and decreasing variability and eventually a prolonged and smooth deceleration (actual tracings).

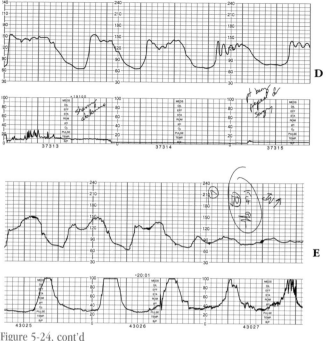

Figure 5-24, cont'd
For legend, see opposite page.

Progression and grading of variable decelerations

Progression of variable decelerations is more important than absolute parameters in distinguishing those that are reassuring from those that are nonreassuring (ACOG, 1995). For example, a *mild variable deceleration* is considered to be one that decelerates to any level for less than 30 seconds because it is very abrupt in both onset and return to baseline. This is considered a variable deceleration with reassuring parameters. When variable decelerations become persistent, progressively deeper, and longer lasting with a prolonged return to baseline, they are considered to have nonreassuring parameters. For example, a *severe variable deceleration* is below 70 bpm for longer than 60 seconds with a slow

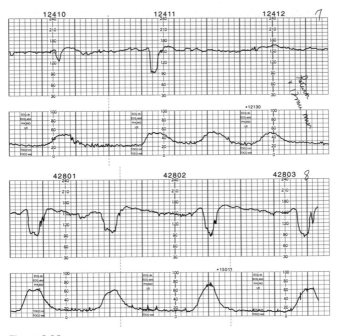

Figure 5-25
Shouldering and overshoots associated with variable
decelerations.

return to baseline. The progressively prolonged return to baseline
is of concern because it reflects the development and progression
of hypoxemia (Freeman et al, 2003). Severe variable decelerations
may also be accompanied by an increase in baseline rate with a
decrease in baseline variability.

Variable decelerations have been graded on the basis of
the depth of the nadir and the duration of the decelerations
(Kubli et al, 1969). However, these are rough quantitative estima-
tions of the severity of variable decelerations. Other parameters,
such as an increase or decrease in baseline rate, or diminishing
or absent variability, are not considered (Freeman et al, 2003).
The grading is based on the duration of the nadir of the variable
decelerations.

NOTE: Grading of variable decelerations is a useful tool in assessing the FHR tracing for any progression in the duration and nadir of variable decelerations. *To fully evaluate the severity of variable decelerations, however, the baseline rate and variability must be assessed.*

Grade of Variable Deceleration	Duration of Nadir
Mild	Any level for <30 sec, regardless of depth, *or* 70 to 80 bpm for <60 sec, *or* >80 bpm for any duration
Moderate	<70 bpm for 30 to 60 sec *or* 70 to 80 bpm for >60 sec
Severe	<70 bpm for >60 sec

Variable decelerations are frequently seen during the second stage of labor and are associated with stretching of the umbilical cord or compression of the cord as the fetus descends through the birth canal. Generally, these decelerations can be tolerated by the fetus if the total time is short from the onset of the decelerations to the time of delivery, as long as the baseline rate is not rising and variability is maintained (Freeman et al, 2003).

A progressively slower return to baseline with repetitive severe variable decelerations indicates a gradual increase in hypoxemia. Severe uncorrectable variable decelerations, particularly with loss of variability and a rise in baseline rate, are associated with fetal hypoxemia, acidemia, and a neurologically depressed newborn.

The following chart summarizes and contrasts reassuring and nonreassuring variable decelerations (Freeman et al, 2003).

Parameters	Reassuring Variable Decelerations	Nonreassuring Variable Decelerations
Time	Less than 30 to 45 sec	<70 bpm for >60 sec
Return to baseline	Rapid, abrupt return to baseline	Prolonged return to baseline, with or without overshoots
Baseline rate	Normal rate continues; does not decrease	Increasing baseline rate
Variability	Moderate variability present; not absent or minimal	Absence of variability

Intervention for Variable Decelerations

Procedure	Rationale
1. Change maternal position from side to side or knee to chest	1. May relieve cord compression
2. When decelerations are severe,	2. Pattern may be a warning or nonreassuring sign
a. Discontinue oxytocin if infusing, remove uterotonic agents; consider tocolytic agents (ACOG, 1995)	a. Decrease any uterine activity that may contribute to cord compression.
b. Administer oxygen 8-10 L at 100% by facemask	b. Hyperoxygenation of maternal blood will increase oxygen saturation of hemoglobin, with maximum increase after 8 to 9 min of 100% oxygen to the woman (McNamara et al, 1993).
c. Vaginal or speculum examination	c. Assess for prolapsed umbilical cord or imminent delivery.
d. Amnioinfusion, especially in the presence of documented oligohy-dramnios (p. 189)	d. Instillation of normal saline or lactated Ringer's solution through the IUPC may decrease frequency and severity of variable decelerations and relieve cord compression.
e. Fetal pulse oximetry may be considered (p. 175).	e. Provides additional data; distinguishes normoxia from hypoxemia in fetus.
f. Prepare for delivery of fetus. Consider if variable deceleration pattern cannot be corrected.	f. Continuation of severe variable decelerations can only further compromise fetal condition by increasing hypoxemia and acidemia.

Summary of Decelerations

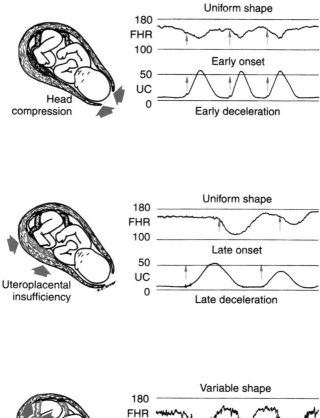

Uniform shape

180
FHR
100

Early onset

50
UC
0

Head
compression

Early deceleration

Uniform shape

180
FHR
100

Late onset

50
UC
0

Uteroplacental
insufficiency

Late deceleration

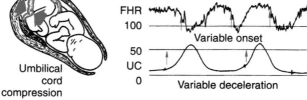

Variable shape

180
FHR
100

Variable onset

50
UC
0

Umbilical
cord
compression

Variable deceleration

	Early Decelerations
ETIOLOGY	Head compression, decrease in cerebral blood flow, vagal response
ONSET	Early and gradual; before peak of UC; uniform and gradual in shape
RECOVERY	By end of contraction, as uterine pressure returns to resting tone; gradual
DECELERATION	Rarely decelerates below 110 bpm, or 30 bpm below baseline
CLINICAL SIGNIFICANCE	Compensatory
NURSING INTERVENTION	Observe for changes of pattern, rate, and variability

Late Decelerations	Variable Decelerations
Uteroplacental insufficiency	Any interruption in umbilical cord blood flow; cord compression
Late, gradual; at or after peak (acme) of UC, nadir (lowest point) well after acme of UC, uniform and gradual in shape	Varies; abrupt; anytime between or during contractions
After the completion of the UC, well after pressure has returned to resting tone	Varies; may have rapid and abrupt return, shouldering over baseline, or a prolonged return with or without overshoot
Nadir usually within the normal FHR range of 110 to 160, may decelerate 30 bpm or more below baseline FHR	Often decelerates with nadir below the normal FHR range
Nonreassuring; requires intervention and treatment	May be mild and reassuring; may progress to nonreassuring with loss of variability, prolonged return to baseline, and increasing baseline rate or tachycardia
Change maternal position.	Change maternal position.
Correct maternal hypotension; elevate legs; increase circulating volume with IV bolus.	If variables are moderate to severe,
Discontinue oxytocic or remove uterotonic medication from birth canal.	Discontinue oxytocic or remove uterotonic medication from birth canal.
Administer oxygen by facemask at 8-10 L/min.	Administer oxygen 8-10 L/min with facemask.
Perform scalp stimulation (not during UC or decelerations).	Perform vaginal or speculum examination to rule out prolapsed cord.
Consider fetal pulse oximetry for additional data.	Consider fetal pulse oximetry for additional data.
Prepare for delivery as indicated.	Perform amnioinfusion.
	Termination of labor may be indicated.

Prolonged Deceleration

Definition

Prolonged deceleration of the fetal heart rate is a visually apparent decrease in FHR to below the baseline. The decrease is determined from the most recently determined portion of the baseline. The decrease from the baseline is more than 15 bpm, lasting more than 2 minutes but less than 10 minutes from onset to return to baseline. A prolonged deceleration of more than 10 minutes is a baseline change (NICHD, 1997).

Description

Generally, a prolonged deceleration is an isolated event. It is most frequently associated with occult or frank cord prolapse, progressive severe variable decelerations, or a profound change in the intrauterine environment. It is characterized by a prolonged deceleration of 2 minutes or more and frequently decelerates to below the average FHR range, although a tachycardic fetus may decelerate within the normal FHR range.

Characteristics (Figure 5-26)

SHAPE	Variable in shape; does not reflect the shape of any associated UC
ONSET	Variable times in the contracting phase
RECOVERY	May last 2 min or more, with a loss of variability and rebound tachycardia; occasionally a period of late decelerations follows; some fetuses do not recover—characterized by a terminal bradycardia and subsequent death.
DECELERATION	Deceleration is almost always below the normal FHR range, except in a fetus with tachycardia.
BASELINE AND VARIABILITY	Often associated with a loss of variability and postdeceleration tachycardia
	May be associated with marked variability after FHR recovers to former baseline rate
OCCURRENCE	Usually isolated events but may be seen during epidural anesthesia, maternal hypotension, late in the course of repetitive severe variable decelerations, during a prolonged series of late decelerations, or with profound change in the intrauterine environment (e.g., maternal seizure, respiratory arrest) before fetal death

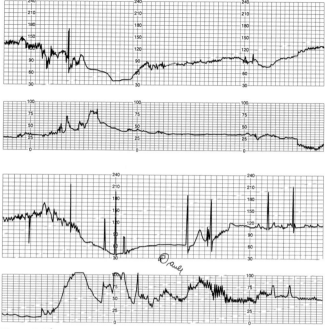

Figure 5-26
Prolonged deceleration.

Etiology

Cause of Prolonged Decelerations	Mechanism
Cord compression (Figure 5-27)	A sudden occult or frank prolapse of the umbilical cord
Maternal hypotension (supine or related to regional anesthesia)	Profound uteroplacental insufficiency may result from hypotension, causing prolonged deceleration.
Paracervical anesthesia	Possibly related to fetal uptake of anesthetic agent, local hypotension from uterine artery spasm, or uterine hypertonus

Cause of Prolonged Decelerations	Mechanism
Tetanic UCs (may be a result of oxytocin stimulation, abruptio placentae, epidural block, breast hyper-stimulation, or cocaine ingestion)	Uterine tetany results in uteroplacental insufficiency; cocaine ingestion can result in vasospasm, hypertonus, and abruption; inadvertent IV injection of anesthetic with epidural block can result in tetanic contraction and prolonged deceleration.
Maternal hypoxemia	Maternal seizure activity or respiratory depression (from narcotic overdose, magnesium sulfate toxicity, or high spinal anesthetic)
Procedures and physiol-ogical mechanisms (e.g., spiral electrode application, pelvic examination, sustained maternal Valsalva, rapid fetal descent through birth canal)	Fetal head compression/stimulation can produce a strong vagal response, cardiodeceleration, and prolonged deceleration.

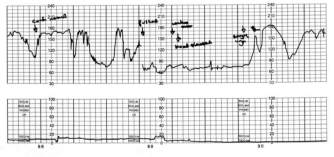

Figure 5-27
Prolonged deceleration due to prolapsed umbilical cord.

Clinical Significance

Prolonged decelerations associated with a vagal response from a procedure (spiral electrode application, pelvic examination), sustained maternal Valsalva, or rapid fetal descent usually last for only 2 minutes and recover with predeceleration variability and baseline. Decelerations caused by maternal hypotension, tetanic contractions, and maternal hypoxemia may be accompanied by a loss of variability and a "rebound" tachycardia or recurrent late decelerations (Figure 5-28). If a subsequent prolonged deceleration does not recur, the placenta generally recovers the fetus to its predeceleration state. *Recovery* is defined as the return of the FHR tracing to the predeceleration state. That is, variability, baseline, and accelerations (if they were present prior to the incident causing the prolonged deceleration) all appear exactly as they did prior to the insult that caused the deceleration.

The prognosis for fetal survival is guarded if the prolonged deceleration occurs after a series of repetitive severe variable decelerations. In this situation, prolonged deceleration and/or

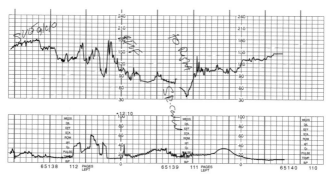

Figure 5-28

Prolonged deceleration following uterine rupture. This deceleration was followed by variable decelerations, fetal tachycardia, and a decrease in variability prior to cesarean delivery. Entire scar from previous cesarean delivery had ruptured and extended into the cervix. The neonate's Apgar scores were 8 at 1 and 9 at 5 minutes.

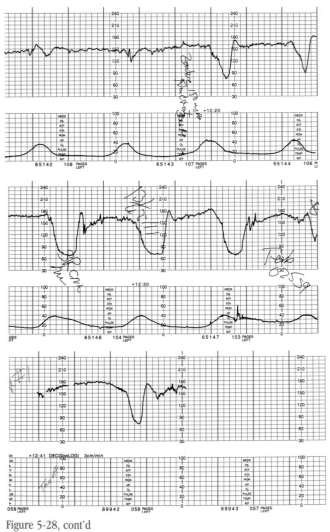

Figure 5-28, cont'd
For legend, see previous page.

recurrent late decelerations may result in a terminal bradycardia of 30 to 60 bpm before fetal death.

Intervention

Intervention is based on identifying and alleviating the cause of the prolonged deceleration. If the apparent cause is severe uteroplacental insufficiency or umbilical cord compression or is unidentifiable, then expeditious delivery may be indicated. Measures used to treat nonreassuring fetal status can be instituted in any case. These measures are described in detail in Chapter 6.

References

American College of Obstetricians and Gynecologists (ACOG): Fetal heart rate patterns: Monitoring, interpretation, and management, *Technical Bulletin* no. 207, Washington, DC, July 1995, The College.

Association of Women's Health, Obstetric, and Neonatal Nurses (AWHONN): *Fetal heart monitoring: Principles and practices*, ed 3, Iowa, 2003, Kendall/Hunt.

Chez BF: *EFM terminology: Communicating if you are reassured or not*, Proceedings of the 3rd annual National Conference of Electronic Fetal Monitoring: The science, the art, the future, Washington, DC, Oct, 1992.

Clinical Effectiveness Support Unit of RCOG: The use of electronic fetal monitoring: The use and interpretation of cardiotography in intrapartum fetal surveillance, *Evidence-based Clinical Guideline* no. 8, London, 2001, Royal College of Obstetricians and Gynecologists (RCOG).

Freeman RK, Garite TJ, Nageotte MP: *Fetal heart rate monitoring*, Baltimore, 2003, Williams & Wilkins.

Garite TJ: Intrapartum fetal evaluation. In Gabbe SG, Niebyl JR, Simpson JL, editors: *Obstetrics: Normal and problem pregnancies*, ed 4, New York, 2002, Churchill Livingstone.

Gilbert ES, Harmon JS: *Manual of high risk pregnancy & delivery*, ed 3, St Louis, 2003, Mosby.

Kleinman CS, Nehgme R, Copel JA: Fetal cardiac arrhythmias: Diagnosis and therapy. In Creasy RK, Resnik R, editors: *Maternal–fetal medicine*, ed 4, Philadelphia, 1999, Saunders.

Kubli FW, Hon EH, Khazin AF, Takemura H: Observations on heart rate and pH in the human fetus during labor, *Am J Obstet Gynecol* 104(8):1190-1206, 1969.

McNamara H, Johnson, Lilford R: The effect on fetal arteriolar oxygen saturation resulting from giving oxygen to the mother measured by pulse oximetry, *Br J Obstet Gynaecol* 100(5):446-449, 1993.

Martin EJ: *Intrapartum management modules: A perinatal educational program*, ed 3, Philadelphia, 2002, Lippincott.

National Institute of Child Health and Human Development (NICHD) Research Planning Workshop: Electronic fetal heart rate monitoring: Research guidelines for interpretation, *Am J Obstet Gynecol* 177(6):1385-1390, 1997.

Parer JT: *Handbook of fetal heart rate monitoring*, Philadelphia, 1997, Saunders.

Simpson KR, Creehan PA: *Perinatal nursing*, ed 2, Philadelphia, 2002, Lippincott.

Assessment and Management of Fetal Status

6

Clinical fetal heart rate (FHR) monitoring is a tool that allows perinatal providers an ongoing observation of fetal physiology (Freeman et al, 2003). The focus of electronic intrapartum FHR monitoring is to screen for fetal well-being, and electronic monitoring is often the primary screening technique for the clinical determination of the adequacy of fetal oxygenation during labor (Parer, 1997). Knowledge of the patterns considered "reassuring," "concerning," and "nonreassuring" is essential to the implementation of appropriate physiological interventions. Because fetal heart rate characteristics reflect acidemia, they also provide information about fetal acid–base status (King, Parer, 2000).

The terms *fetal stress* and *fetal distress* have been replaced with the term *nonreassuring fetal status*. *Fetal distress* is an imprecise term that includes far more than an interpretation of fetal heart rate characteristics. *Nonreassuring fetal status* is a descriptive term that is used when the clinician who is interpreting the data is not reassured by the findings (ACOG, 1998; RCOG, 2001). The nonreassuring findings consist of a loss of variability that may be accompanied by a change in baseline rate and may include the appearance of periodic and episodic patterns (severe variable decelerations, late decelerations, or a bradycardia) that persist despite interventions. The presence of FHR variability indicates central nervous system and myocardial normoxia, whereas its decrease or absence in the presence of decelerations or bradycardia indicates a decrease in oxygenation to the CNS and myocardium (Parer, 1997). Diminished variability is secondary to a breakdown in the fetal compensatory mechanism to remain oxygenated. A progression to decreased, exaggerated (marked), or absent baseline variability or a sinusoidal pattern may occur and, without intervention or delivery, may lead to fetal morbidity or mortality.

Research and experience suggest that a previously "normoxic" term fetus (without risk factors such as intrauterine growth restriction or oligohydramnios) can tolerate late or severe variable decelerations for approximately 30 minutes before showing signs of decompensation when variability remains present (Parer, 1997). It is crucial for all members of the obstetrical care delivery team to formulate and agree on a plan of action for intervention before the end of a 30-minute period of nonreassuring FHR tracing that has not been corrected or shown improvement as a result of interventions to enhance and optimize uteroplacental blood flow and fetal oxygenation.

Literature and practice indicate that an abnormal electronic fetal monitoring tracing is a poor predictor of cerebral palsy (CP). In reality, (1) electronic fetal monitoring has failed to detect severe fetal asphyxia in an undetermined number of cases, (2) perinatal asphyxia is an uncommon cause of CP (possible causes include congenital developmental defects, intrauterine growth restriction, coagulation and autoimmune disorders, intrauterine infection, intrauterine exposure to toxins and teratogens, trauma, and neonatal asphyxia [Hankins, 1991]), and (3) electronic fetal monitoring patterns that reflect fetal asphyxia or acidosis may be the result of a damaged fetal brain and may be a consequence, instead of the cause, of CP (MacLennan, 1999).

An evidence-based report issued by the American College of Obstetricians and Gynecologists (ACOG) and the American Academy of Pediatrics (AAP), "Neonatal Encephalopathy and Cerebral Palsy: Defining the Pathogenesis and Pathophysiology" (2003), and an earlier report, "A Template for Defining a Causal Relation Between Intrapartum Events and Cerebral Palsy: International Consensus Statement" (MacLennan, 1999), both highlight the rarity with which acute intrapartum events are associated with cerebral palsy. Other causes of cerebral palsy that are identified in these reports include a set of criteria that identify whether an acute hypoxemic intrapartum event has contributed to neonatal brain injury. Further discussion is found in Chapter 1.

As assessment tools are used and studied, a better understanding of the fetal response to stress (e.g., uterine contractions) has resulted. Literature and practitioners continue to disagree on the validity, efficacy, and cost effectiveness of surveillance tools and methods. This is in part the result of a lack of agreement about some definitions, labels, and parameters that warrant intervention. It is recommended that a chain of command and a plan be developed and agreed on by the obstetrical medical, anesthetic, neonatal/pediatric, nursing, and hospital administration staff for interventions for nonreassuring FHR patterns well before intervention is necessary (see Chapter 11, Figure 11-1). This consultation plan should be based on accepted standards of practice for the level of care provided in the institution, on resources, and on personnel available in each care setting.

In conclusion, the focus of assessment of a fetal monitoring tracing is to identify patterns that are reassuring and predictive of a positive fetal outcome, as well as those that are nonreassuring, in order to provide appropriate interventions. This chapter discusses reassuring and nonreassuring patterns, interventions, and adjuncts to fetal assessment.

Assessment of Fetal Status

The modality used (i.e., external or internal monitoring) and the frequency of assessment of fetal status should be guided by the risk status of both the mother and the fetus. There is no evidence-based difference in perinatal outcome between continuous fetal monitoring and intermittent auscultation. The standards of practice and guidelines for patient care and frequency of evaluating and recording fetal status during the intrapartum period are outlined in the following chart (Simpson, Creehan, 2001; AAP/ACOG, 2002; AWHONN, 2003).

Frequency of Assessing Fetal Heart Rate

Stage of Labor	Low Risk	High Risk
Active Phase*	q 30 minutes	q 15 minutes
Second Stage	q 15 minutes	q 5 minutes
Auscultated FHR	Determine and record the auscultated FHR just after a contraction at the prescribed intervals.	
Electronically monitored FHR	Evaluate tracing at the prescribed intervals.	

* Latent phase: See p. 39.

The process of assessing fetal status during both the intrapartum and the antepartum periods should be done in a thorough and systematic manner. The baseline FHR should be identified as being within the normal FHR range, tachycardia, or bradycardia.

The amplitude of baseline variability should be assessed, noting the presence or absence of short-term variability, when a fetal spiral electrode is in place. Periodic changes associated with uterine contractions and episodic or spontaneous changes should be noted, including accelerations and early, late, variable, or prolonged decelerations. Uterine activity should be assessed for the frequency and duration of contractions, and, if the woman is monitored by manual palpation, the strength and resting tone should be noted. For women being monitored internally with an intrauterine pressure catheter (IUPC), the intensity and resting tone in millimeters of mercury (mm Hg) pressure or Montevideo units (MVU) should be assessed. The following checklist is a tool that can be used to evaluate the FHR and uterine activity on a monitor tracing.

CHECKLIST FOR ASSESSMENT OF FETAL HEART RATE AND UTERINE ACTIVITY

1. What is the baseline fetal heart rate (FHR)?
   _____ Beats per minute (bpm)
   Check one of the following as observed on the tracing/monitor strip:
   _____ Average baseline FHR (normal range of 110 to 160 bpm)
   _____ Tachycardia (>160 bpm)
   _____ Bradycardia (<110 bpm)
2. What is the baseline variability?
   _____ Absent (range undetectable)
   _____ Minimal (just detectable to ≤5 bpm)
   _____ Moderate (6 to 25 bpm)
   _____ Marked (>25 bpm)
   _____ Short-term variability: absent or present
   _____ Undulating baseline
3. Are there any changes in the FHR? (1) Periodic—associated with uterine contractions, or (2) Episodic—spontaneous.
   _____ Accelerations; spontaneous, with fetal movement or stimulation
   _____ Accelerations with uterine contractions
   _____ Early decelerations (head compression)
   _____ Late decelerations (uteroplacental insufficiency)
   _____ Variable decelerations (cord compression)
      _____ Reassuring (<30 to 45 seconds, abrupt return to baseline, normal baseline rate, moderate variability)

_____ Nonreassuring (>60 seconds, slow return to baseline, increasing baseline rate, absence of variability)

_____ Prolonged deceleration (>15 bpm below baseline, >2 minutes to <10 minutes)

4. What is the uterine activity/contraction pattern (UA/UC)?

_____ Frequency (onset to onset of UC)

_____ Duration (beginning to end of contraction)

Abdominal palpation method

_____ Strength: mild, moderate, or strong

_____ Resting time: from end of UC to start of next UC

Internal monitoring/intrauterine pressure catheter

_____ Intensity in mm Hg

_____ Resting tone in mm Hg

Reassuring Fetal Heart Rate Patterns

A reassuring fetal heart rate pattern (Figure 6-1) is one that confers an extremely high predictability of a normally oxygenated fetus at the time it is obtained. The following parameters reflect a reassuring fetal heart rate (NICHD, 1997).

Baseline rate	110 to 160 bpm
Variability	Moderate ≥6 to ≤25 bpm
Periodic/episodic changes	Presence of accelerations, absence of decelerations

NOTE: Early decelerations and reassuring variable decelerations are not concerning but must be observed for any changes in pattern.

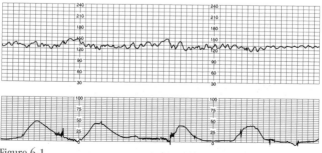

Figure 6-1
Reassuring FHR and uterine activity pattern.

Normal Uterine Contraction Pattern

The following parameters for normal uterine contraction frequency, duration intensity and resting tone follow:

FREQUENCY	More than 2 minutes from the start of one contraction to the next
DURATION	Less than 90 seconds from onset to end of contraction
INTENSITY	Less than 80 mm Hg pressure in the first stage of labor
RESTING TONE	Intrauterine pressure less than 20 mm Hg depending on type of IUPC; 30 seconds or more between contractions

NOTE: Resting tone may be slightly higher if labor is being augmented or induced with an oxytocic agent.

The presence of a normal, or reassuring, FHR and uterine activity pattern serves to allay the concerns of the woman and staff about the fetal status during labor. A reassuring pattern is reliably predictive of fetal tolerance of labor, normal oxygen and acid–base status, and vigor at birth (ACOG, 1995a).

Concerning Fetal Heart Rate Patterns

Concerning FHR patterns may be self-limiting or they may progress to nonreassuring FHR patterns. If the recording of these patterns is not clear or is of poor quality, or if a more accurate assessment of the pattern is necessary, the direct method of monitoring with a spiral electrode should be considered until the pattern becomes reassuring or until intervention for a nonreassuring pattern is indicated. Concerning patterns include the following:

- Progressive increase/decrease or shift in baseline FHR
- Tachycardia of 160 bpm or more
- Decreasing baseline variability without any identified cause (such as narcotics, sleep cycle)

Nonreassuring Fetal Heart Rate Patterns and Interventions (see Table 6-1, p. 168)

Nonreassuring FHR patterns (Figures 6-2 to 6-4) are those characterized by specific periodic and episodic FHR changes, loss of variability, and bradycardia. Identification of these patterns is important to provide appropriate cause-specific interventions.

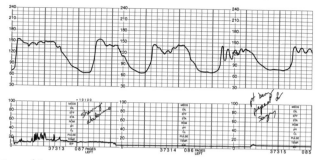

Figure 6-2

Nonreassuring FHR pattern: severe variable decelerations with a decreasing baseline rate, minimal variability, and undulations of baseline in the last 3 minutes of the tracing.

Nonreassuring patterns include the following:

- Severe variable decelerations with FHR nadir below 70 bpm, for more than 60 seconds, with any of the following:
  - Rising baseline rate
  - Decreasing variability
  - Slow return to baseline
- Late decelerations, more serious if associated with the following:
  - Decreasing variability
  - Rising baseline rate
- Absence of variability
- Prolonged deceleration
- Severe bradycardia
- Sinusoidal pattern

Nonreassuring FHR patterns predictive of current or impending fetal asphyxia of such severity that the fetus is at risk of neurological and other fetal damage or death (NICHD, 1997) include the following:

- Recurrent late decelerations with absent FHR variability
- Recurrent variable decelerations with absent FHR variability
- Substantial bradycardia with absent FHR variability

Nonreassuring fetal heart rate patterns are associated with metabolic, respiratory, or mixed acidosis, and when uncorrected they may lead to fetal morbidity or mortality. The primary goal of interventions is to optimize and enhance fetal oxygenation, as reflected by conversion to a reassuring FHR pattern. The physiological goals

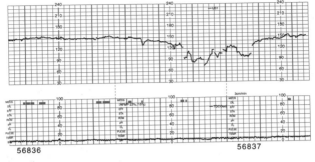

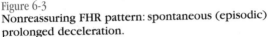

Figure 6-3
Nonreassuring FHR pattern: spontaneous (episodic)
prolonged deceleration.

of the interventions are intended to maximize uterine blood flow, umbilical circulation, and oxygenation, and to reduce uterine activity (AWHONN, 2003). The conventional interventions used for *intrauterine resuscitation* include maternal position change, hydration, maternal oxygen administration, a decrease or discontinuance of uterine stimulant medications, and provider notification. Cause-specific interventions based on the type of nonreassuring pattern, along with their purposes and rationales, are described in Table 6-1. When efforts fail to convert the fetal status to a reassuring one, the interventions should continue to optimize fetal oxygenation until delivery is effected. Other interventions that may improve the FHR pattern include amnioinfusion to ameliorate variable decelerations, and tocolytic medications to reduce uterine activity.

Mixed fetal heart rate patterns should be evaluated by the most nonreassuring component of the pattern, such as absent baseline variability or late decelerations.

NOTE: The most nonreassuring component provides the direction for appropriate interventions.

Mixed or combination fetal heart rate patterns include the following:

■ Early and variable decelerations
■ Early and late decelerations
■ Late and variable decelerations
■ Prolonged deceleration following any other deceleration

Although electronic fetal monitoring was intended to be used as a reflector of the adequacy of fetal oxygenation and not to reflect brain

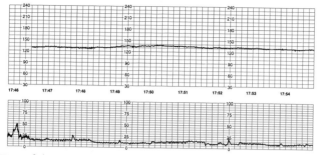

Figure 6-4
Nonreassuring pattern: absence of variability.

function, some FHR patterns have been described as usually consistent with existing fetal brain damage. These include the following:

- A flat tracing without late decelerations, variable decelerations, or prolonged bradycardia has been described with anencephaly (Dicker et al, 1983; Van der Moer et al, 1985).
- A wandering pattern of blunt, slow, irregular undulations with a flat baseline has been reported with anencephaly (Freeman et al, 2003).
- A sinusoidal electronic fetal monitoring pattern has been described in cases of hydrocephalus and severe anemia (Ombelet, Van der Moer, 1985; Parer, 1997).
- A fixed heart rate with late decelerations and terminal bradycardias has been reported to occur in fetuses with severe CNS anomalies (Didolkar, Mutch, 1979).

Preterminal patterns may include any of the following: total loss of variability; rounded, blunted-appearing decelerations that resemble severe variable decelerations; an unstable wandering baseline; fetal tachycardia; a sinusoidal pattern; a fixed heart rate with a flat baseline; and a profound bradycardia preceding the terminal event (Figure 6-5). These patterns may also be seen in fetuses with major congenital anomalies (Freeman et al, 2003).

For predicting neonatal outcome, a nonreassuring fetal heart rate pattern lacks the reliability of a reassuring pattern; that is, the nonreassuring FHR pattern is not necessarily predictive of whether the fetus will be well oxygenated, depressed, or acidotic (ACOG, 1995a). A reason for the unreliability of the nonreassuring FHR pattern is that most fetuses respond to cause-specific interventions

Text continued on p. 172

Table 6-1   Identification and management of nonreassuring fetal heart rate (FHR) patterns

Nonreassuring FHR Patterns	Intervention

Severe variable deceleration
  FHR nadir below 70 bpm,
  lasting longer than 60 seconds
  with any of the following:
  ■ Rising baseline FHR
  ■ Decreasing variability
  ■ Slow return to baseline
	a. Change maternal position
	
	b. Evaluate for trends, changes in baseline rate, and variability
	c. Perform vaginal examination
	
	d. No scalp stimulation with deceleration nadir
	e. Remove uterotonic agents if hyperstimulation is occurring
	
	f. Administer oxygen at 8-10 L/min at 100% by facemask
	g. Amnioinfusion may be considered
	
	h. Increase rate of maintenance IV infusion (bolus)
	
	i. Fetal pulse oximetry may be considered*
	j. Tocolytic agents and termination of labor should be considered if pattern cannot be corrected enough to meet criteria of mild deceleration; prepare for delivery

*Consider when fetus meets criteria for class II nonreassuring fetal status (see Table 6-2, p. 176).

Purpose	Rationale
a. To relieve pressure on the umbilical cord	a. Improves and optimizes umbilical and uteroplacental blood flow
b. To identify increasing FHR, decreasing variability, or slowing return to baseline	b. Indicates progressive deterioration of FHR pattern
c. To rule out a prolapsed cord, rapid descent, or imminent delivery	c. Continue other interventions or prepare for emergent cesarean delivery if cord is prolapsed
d. To reduce repetitive pressure on cord	d. Avoids additional stress to fetus
e. To decrease uterine hyperstimulation	e. Decreases strength and frequency of uterine contractions (which contribute to cord compression)
f. To promote maternal hyperoxia	f. Maximizes fetal oxygenation
g. To relieve pressure on umbilical cord by adding fluid to cushion cord	g. Corrects oligohydramnios and maximizes umbilical circulation
h. To correct maternal hypotension and reverse dehydration	h. Increases circulating volume, maximizes oxygenation and uteroplacental perfusion
i. To distinguish normoxia from hypoxemia in the fetus	i. A value less than 30% indicates hypoxemia
j. To decrease stress on or hypoxemia in fetus	j. Fetal position, stage of labor, and dilatation should be considered if labor continues in the presence of a nonreassuring FHR pattern

Continued

Table 6-1   Identification and management of nonreassuring
fetal heart rate (FHR) patterns—cont'd

Nonreassuring FHR Patterns	Intervention
Late decelerations of any magnitude are more serious if associated with either of the following: ■ Decreasing variability ■ Rising baseline	Intervene with step-by-step approach, proceeding from one step to the next if pattern is uncorrected 1. Place patient in lateral position 2. Lower head of bed 3. Increase rate of maintenance IV infusion 4. Discontinue oxytocin if infusing (do this first if uterine hyperstimulation is present); consider tocolysis 5. Administer oxygen at 10 L/min at 100% via facemask 6. Consider fetal pulse oximetry*
Absence of variability Prolonged deceleration Severe bradycardia Sinusoidal pattern	Correct identifiable cause; administer maternal oxygen; consider fetal pulse oximetry†

NOTE: See discussion of tocolysis therapy for nonreassuring FHR patterns (under
Intrapartal Tocolysis Therapy for Nonreassuring FHR Patterns).
*Consider when fetus meets criteria for class II nonreassuring fetal status.

Purpose	Rationale
1. To correct supine hypotension and improve uterine blood flow	1. Removes the weight of the fetus from the inferior vena cava, which allows better blood return to the heart, increasing maternal cardiac output and subsequently blood pressure, and maximizes uteroplacental perfusion
2. To correct maternal hypotension	2. Diminishes pooling of blood in extremities and increases circulating volume
3. To correct maternal hypotension and reverse dehydration	3. Increases circulating blood volume and uteroplacental perfusion
4. To reduce uterine activity	4. Decreases strength and frequency of uterine contractions, improving uteroplacental blood flow
5. To promote maternal hyperoxia	5. Maximizes fetal oxygenation
6. To distinguish normoxia from hypoxemia	6. Values less than 30% indicate hypoxemia
To determine if pattern results from narcotic administration, maternal position, uterine hyperstimulation, rapid descent, cord prolapse, abruption, uterine rupture, fetal anomaly, or prolonged uteroplacental insufficiency	Identifies a cause that may be reversible or changeable. If it is not, document event, notify appropriate obstetrical team members, prepare for immediate delivery

†Consider when fetus meets criteria for class II nonreassuring fetal status (see Table 6-2, p. 176).

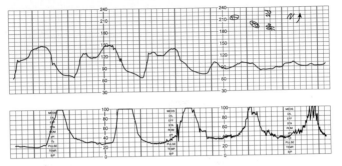

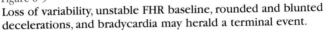

Figure 6-5
Loss of variability, unstable FHR baseline, rounded and blunted decelerations, and bradycardia may herald a terminal event.

(such as changing maternal position for supine hypotension) to correct a nonreassuring pattern to a reassuring one. A reassuring pattern is highly predictive of a well-oxygenated fetus, whereas some fetuses with nonreassuring FHR patterns are not depressed or acidotic and do not have an adverse outcome (Garite, 2002). In other fetuses, nonreassuring patterns may not be related to hypoxia but may be the result of other factors such as congenital neurological abnormalities (e.g., anencephaly).

Other Methods of Assessment

The primary premise for intrapartum surveillance is the timely identification of and intervention for fetal hypoxemia or acidosis. Studies show that most accurate assessments of fetal well-being and degree of acidemia are obtained when electronic fetal monitoring is used in conjunction with other tools. Some tools of assessment are used during the intrapartum period, such as scalp stimulation, and others after delivery, such as cord gases, to reconstruct hypoxemic episodes. To date, fetal pulse oximetry appears to be the optimal method for distinguishing the intrapartum fetus that has a nonreassuring FHR pattern but is adequately oxygenated, from one that is *not* adequately oxygenated.

Fetal Stimulation Tests

Intrapartum stimulation tests are useful to rule out fetal acidemia in the presence of a nonreassuring FHR pattern. Stimulation of the fetus to elicit an acceleration of the FHR is an alternative to scalp pH testing (Skupski et al, 2002). The use of fetal scalp pH in clinical practice has decreased, without negatively impacting the rate of morbidity and mortality in neonates, because of an increase in the use of intrapartum fetal stimulation testing (Goodwin et al, 1994). These tests are for *screening* purposes and are *not* intended to be used as interventions during a deceleration or bradycardia. Stimulation should be done during the "reserve" period of the FHR—that is, between contractions and decelerations.

Procedure

Stimulation methods include the following:

1. *Scalp stimulation:* Digital pressure and stroking of the fetal scalp for 15 seconds during a vaginal examination.
2. *Sound stimulation:* Vibroacoustic stimulation (VAS) by placing an artificial larynx on the maternal abdomen over the fetal head continuously for 3 to 5 seconds. Because amniotic fluid is necessary for the transmission of both sound and vibration, VAS is recommended for use only with intact membranes.

NOTE: Do not perform these procedures during a contraction or FHR deceleration.

Do not perform these procedures in the presence of fetal bradycardia.

Interpretation and clinical significance

The rationale for use of these procedures is that if the stimulation produces an acceleration of 15 bpm for 15 seconds in a fetus beyond 32 weeks of gestational age (or 10 bpm for 10 seconds if the fetus is ≤32 weeks), one can assume that the fetal pH is normal. Several studies have shown a high correlation between fetal heart rate acceleration in response to scalp or sound stimulation and a fetal scalp pH above 7.2. Therefore there is a significantly low likelihood of fetal acidemia in the presence of FHR acceleration. Repeat stimulation during the course of labor may be necessary and is advisable if FHR abnormalities persist (Skupski et al, 2002). Retesting for FHR acceleration every 30 minutes in the continued presence of a nonreassuring pattern should be considered to continue to rule out acidemia.

When there is no FHR acceleration, there is a significantly increased likelihood of fetal acidemia. However, of the fetuses that do not show FHR acceleration, about half are *not* acidemic, so absence of FHR acceleration to the stimulus is not reliably predictive of an abnormal pH and fetal acidosis. In addition, a lack of an acceleratory response may be due to exposure to drugs (CNS depressants, illicit drugs) or to central nervous system injury.

Fetal Blood Sampling for Acid–Base Status

Fetal blood sampling (Figure 6-6) was first described by Saling in 1962 as a means of identifying fetal hypoxemia and acidosis. When the fetus is faced with hypoxia, the metabolism changes from aerobic to anaerobic. This results in the production of lactic acid and a subsequent drop in pH. Therefore a decrease in blood pH becomes a measure of the degree of hypoxemia. Thus fetal scalp sampling was developed as a means of identifying the degree of fetal hypoxemia at the time of testing.

Studies have shown that many variables can lead to false elevations *or* decreases of the pH. These variables can influence the pH during the intrapartum/predelivery period and make values disproportionate to the condition at birth. These factors include the following:

- Maternal acidosis or alkalosis
- Laboratory errors or delay in determination
- Caput succedaneum (↓ pH value)
- Stage of labor
- Time relationship of scalp sampling to uterine contractions
- Influence of in utero treatment

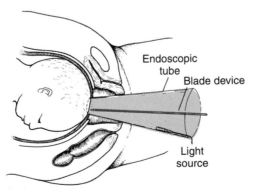

Figure 6-6
Schema of fetal blood sampling.

- Transience of the insult causing fetal acidosis (metabolic acidosis is less readily reversible than respiratory acidosis)
- Contamination of sample with amniotic fluid ($\downarrow$ pH value) or room air ($\uparrow$ pH value)
- Contamination with meconium

Because of the invasive nature of fetal scalp blood sampling, the high rate of inaccurate results, and the delay in obtaining results, this technique is seldom used in perinatal units in the United States (Simpson, 1998). Studies have demonstrated that fetuses with acceleration of the fetal heart rate by scalp or acoustic stimulation reliably rule out acidemia in the presence of nonreassuring FHR patterns. Because of the relative ease of performing scalp or sound stimulation to rule out acidemia, the procedure of scalp pH testing has been virtually replaced.

Fetal Pulse Oximetry

Fetal pulse oximetry monitoring is the most significant change in intrapartum fetal assessment since the introduction of FHR monitoring and fetal scalp sampling almost 40 years ago. The primary value of fetal pulse oximetry is to better assess intrapartum fetal status in the presence of a nonreassuring FHR pattern as observed during electronic FHR monitoring. The value obtained reliably distinguishes the fetus that is adequately oxygenated from the fetus that is not. Information about fetal oxygen saturation ($FSpO_2$) obtained through pulse oximetry provides additional data for a more complete picture of fetal status, which helps to clarify the direction for clinical management—that is, the continuation of labor or the need for intervention.

Intended use for fetal pulse oximetry

As an adjunct to FHR monitoring, initiation of fetal pulse oximetry should be considered when the fetus presents a class II nonreassuring FHR tracing (Table 6-2). Fetal pulse oximetry is *not* intended to be used for class I reassuring FHR patterns or for class III ominous FHR patterns.

Contraindications

Fetal pulse oximetry is to be used as an adjunct to electronic FHR monitoring in the presence of a class II nonreassuring fetal heart rate pattern. It is *not intended* to be used in the

Table 6-2   Classification of fetal heart rate (FHR) patterns: Guide for the use of fetal pulse oximetry

Class I **REASSURING**	Any FHR pattern that does not meet criteria for class II or III. Typically, a class I trace is characterized by a baseline of between 110 and 160 bpm, with long-term variability of between 5 and 25 bpm, and either no decelerations or only early decelerations.

Class II
NONREAS-
SURING*
	Any one of the following for >15 min:
	■ Persistent late decelerations (>50% of contractions)
	■ Sinusoidal pattern[†]
	■ Variable decelerations with one or more of the following:
	  ■ A relative drop of ≥70 bpm or an absolute drop to ≤70 bpm for >60 sec[‡]
	  ■ Persistent slow return to baseline
	  ■ Long-term variability <5 bpm[§]
	  ■ Tachycardia >160 bpm
	■ Recurrent prolonged decelerations (two or more of <70 bpm for >90 sec)
	Either of the following for >60 min:
	■ Tachycardia >160 bpm with long-term variability of <5 bpm[§]
	■ Persistent decreased variability of ≤5 bpm for >60 min[§]

Class III **OMINOUS**	■ Prolonged deceleration to <70 bpm for >7 min[‖] ■ Markedly decreased or absent variability with persistent late decelerations ■ Markedly decreased or absent variability with severe variable decelerations

Reprinted by permission of Nellcor Puritan Bennett, Inc., Pleasanton, Calif.

*Fetal pulse oximetry is indicated for class II nonreassuring patterns only.

[†]Sinusoidal pattern is defined as regular oscillations about the baseline, 5 to 15 bpm in magnitude, with 2 to 5 cycles/min on an otherwise normal baseline with absent short-term variability.

[‡]Variable decelerations are to be timed from the beginning of the deceleration to the end of the deceleration (i.e., >60 sec in duration).

[§]Decreased variability not otherwise explained by the clinical situation (e.g., due to narcotic administration).

[‖]It is not necessary to wait for >7 min of prolonged deceleration before initiating intervention (e.g., evaluation of the cause, nonsurgical intervention, and preparation for delivery), even with reassuring $FSpO_2$.

following situations:

1. In the presence of a reassuring (class I) FHR tracing
2. In the presence of an ominous (class III) FHR pattern as defined in the FHR classification list (see Table 6-2)
3. When the woman is not in active labor
4. When membranes are intact/unruptured
5. In the presence of documented or suspected placenta previa
6. When the woman is seropositive for HIV, hepatitis B, or hepatitis E
7. When the woman has active genital herpes or any other infection that precludes internal monitoring
8. When the pregnancy is less than 36 weeks of gestation
9. In the case of a multiple gestation pregnancy (twins, triplets, or other multiples)
10. When there is a need for immediate delivery (not related to FHR tracing) (e.g., active uterine bleeding)

Description and mechanism of pulse oximetry technology

The fetal pulse oximeter measures functional oxygen saturation of arterial hemoglobin ($FSpO_2$) and the Nellcor monitor detects the fetal pulse rate via a flexible-tipped reflectance sensor positioned against the fetal cheek. The technique of placement is similar to that used for an IUPC and is described in more detail later. In an oximeter used for nonfetal patients, the optical components are found on opposite sides of the monitoring surface, but the fetal oximeter differs in that it uses a reflectance sensor in which the optical components are on the same monitoring surface. The light-emitting diodes (LEDs) on the sensor shine light into tissue, and the photodetector measures the back-scattered light—that is, the reflection of light coming *out* of the tissue (Figure 6-7).

The same basic principles of physics apply to both conventional (extrauterine) and fetal pulse oximetry. However, in fetal oximetry a unique calibration matrix and a different wavelength for the sensor's red LED are used to optimize monitoring in the relatively low range of oxygen saturation values seen in the fetus. Typically, $FSpO_2$ is between 30% and 70% during labor, whereas the saturation of the extrauterine patient is generally 95% to 100% (Figure 6-8).

Pulse oximetry takes advantage of the fact that well-oxygenated blood looks bright red in comparison to poorly oxygenated blood. The fetal sensor contains two LEDs of different wavelengths (Figure 6-9): one red (735 nm) and one infrared (890 nm). The red

Transmission sensor

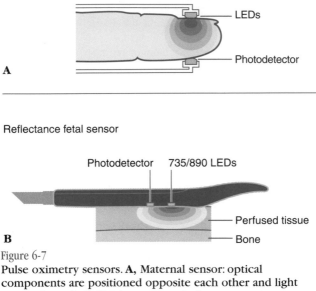

A

Reflectance fetal sensor

B

Figure 6-7
Pulse oximetry sensors. **A,** Maternal sensor: optical components are positioned opposite each other and light passes through. **B,** Fetal sensor: optical components are positioned on the same side and light is reflected back from the tissue.
(Reprinted by permission of Nellcor Puritan Bennett, Inc., Pleasanton, Calif.)

light is absorbed more by deoxyhemoglobin (dark blood), and the infrared light is absorbed more by oxyhemoglobin (bright red blood). The photodetector captures the light that is reflected back from the blood in the tissues of the fetal cheek. The difference between the amount of light that is emitted by the LEDs and the amount that is reflected back represents the amount of light that is absorbed by both oxyhemoglobin and deoxyhemoglobin. It is this difference that is used in the determination of fetal oxygen saturation. The greater the ratio of red to infrared, the lower the oxygen saturation, and vice versa (Dildy et al, 1996).

Monitoring equipment

The Nellcor fetal pulse oximetry system (OxiFirst Fetal Pulse Oximetry system [including the N-400 monitor and fetal sensor], Pleasanton, Calif.) is currently the only system that has undergone

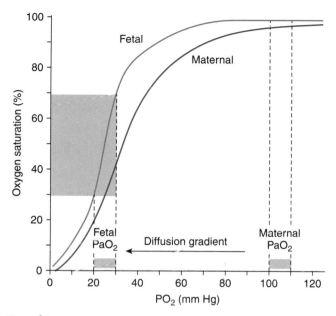

Figure 6-8
Fetal/adult oxyhemoglobin dissociation curves. A fetal PO_2 at the placental interface of 20 to 30 mm Hg corresponds to an $FSpO_2$ of 30% to 70%.
(Reprinted by permission of Nellcor Puritan Bennett, Inc., Pleasanton, Calif.)

multicenter, randomized, controlled clinical trials in the United States. The Nellcor FS-14 Series Fetal Oxygen Sensor (Figure 6-10) can be used only with the OxiFirst system (Figure 6-11) or with an electronic fetal monitor containing patented Nellcor technology. Fetal monitors containing the integrated Nellcor technology include the Philips Medical Products Series 50 XMO monitors (Figure 6-12) and the Corometrics 120 Series fetal monitors (GE Medical Systems Information Technologies, Milwaukee, Wisc.). The fetal sensor plugs into the patient module cable on the face of these fetal monitors, and the fetal oxygen saturation is displayed on the monitor screen and traced on the monitor strip. Through the use of an interface cable, the N-400 stand-alone fetal oximeter can be connected to the aforementioned fetal monitor models if they do not contain the integrated fetal pulse oximetry module, as well as to some older fetal monitors, including the

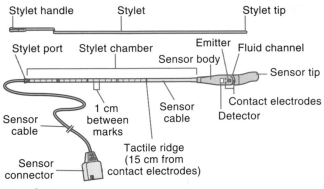

Figure 6-9
Nellcor fetal oxygen sensor (illustration) with key points identified.
(Reprinted by permission of Nellcor Puritan Bennett, Inc., Pleasanton, Calif.)

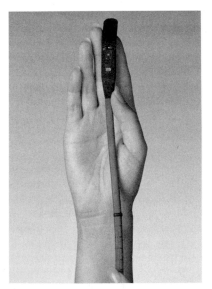

Figure 6-10
Nellcor FS-14 Series fetal oxygen sensor.
(Reprinted by permission of Nellcor Puritan Bennett, Inc., Pleasanton, Calif.)

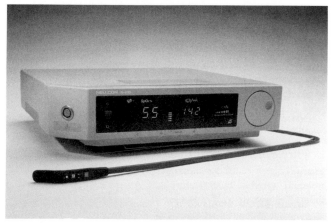

Figure 6-11
The Nellcor N-400 fetal pulse oximeter can interface with a
fetal monitor with a connecting cable. The FSpO$_2$ will trace
on the uterine activity panel of the tracing.
(Reprinted by permission of Nellcor Puritan Bennett, Inc., Pleasanton, Calif.)

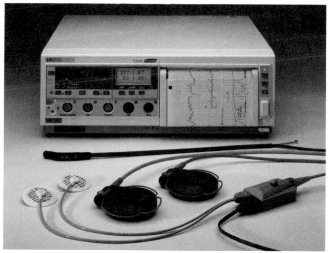

Figure 6-12
Viridia 50XMO fetal maternal monitor with port for Nellcor
Sensor FS-14 to monitor FSpO$_2$.
(Courtesy Philips Medical Systems, Böblingen, Germany.)

Corometrics model 118, Hewlett Packard (HP) model 8040A, Viridia Series 50 IP, and the Meridian Sonicaid 800 monitor.

Whether the fetal pulse oximeter is interfaced with or integrated into the fetal monitor, the technology provides for simultaneous documentation of fetal oxygen saturation, uterine activity, and FHR on the same tracing. Fetal oxygen saturation values are recorded as a line in the uterine activity area of the monitor strip (Figure 6-13). These two parameters are conveniently recorded together because both are measured on a 1- to 100-unit scale.

Requirements for sensor insertion

The following requirements must be met prior to sensor insertion:
1. Presence of a nonreassuring class II FHR pattern (described in Table 6-2)
2. Gestation of 36 weeks or more
3. Singleton fetus
4. Vertex presentation
5. Ruptured membranes
6. Cervix dilated to at least 2 cm
7. Fetal station of −2 or below

NOTE: The sensor may not be used during water births or in any situation where the woman is immersed in water.

Remove the sensor prior to assisted delivery with a vacuum extractor or forceps, and prior to cesarean delivery.

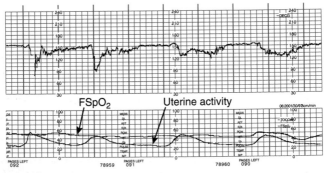

Figure 6-13

Note pulse oximetry tracing on uterine activity panel of fetal monitoring strip.

(Reprinted by permission of Nellcor Puritan Bennett, Inc., Pleasanton, Calif.)

Fetal sensor placement and position

The fetal oximetry sensor, a flexible intrauterine device, is inserted in a manner similar to that of the intrauterine pressure catheter but with some notable differences. Although inserted through the cervical os, the sensor is not advanced into the uterine cavity nearly as far as the IUPC is. The procedure for insertion and placement at the optimal location is a learned skill and should follow the manufacturer's directions. Insertion of the sensor is initiated with an examination of the presenting part. After the sagittal suture and one or both of the fontanels are identified, the sensor is introduced between uterine contractions perpendicular to the sagittal suture and slightly toward the anterior fontanel. Following this procedure allows the fetal oximetry sensor to lie alongside the cheek and temple area of the fetal face (Figure 6-14). This site is optimal for monitoring because fetal pulses tend to be larger in this area, and artifact problems that can be caused by hair, vernix, caput, and venous stasis are not typically encountered. The sensor's fulcrum tip design helps to hold the sensor in place. The fulcrum design allows the sensor tip to flex with the natural forces of labor, thereby taking up any space between the fetal head and the uterine wall. As labor progresses, the sensor generally descends and rotates with the presenting part. On occasion, a minor adjustment to the sensor's position may be required. A complete and detailed description of the sensor placement technique can be found in the manufacturer's clinical use guide.

Critical threshold value for fetal oxygen saturation

The basic interpretation model for fetal oxygen saturation ($FSpO_2$) depends on the existence of a critical threshold value that reliably separates the fetus that is adequately oxygenated from one that is not. The critical threshold is the point below which hypoxemia would cause metabolic acidosis, or above which there would be no risk for acidosis (Garite, Porreco, 2001). Both animal and human studies support the existence of a critical threshold value for fetal oxygen saturation at 30% based on the correlation between fetal oxygen saturation and fetal scalp pH during labor. Kühnert et al. (1998a) found that a fetal saturation of greater than or equal to 30% is predictive of a fetal scalp pH of greater than or equal to 7.20 with 81% sensitivity and 100% specificity. Low fetal arterial oxygen saturation values of less than 30% for 10 minutes or longer

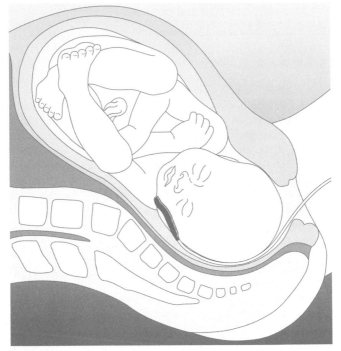

Figure 6-14
Placement and position of fetal oximetry sensor.
(Reprinted by permission of Nellcor Puritan Bennett, Inc., Pleasanton, Calif.)

correlate significantly with low scalp pH values and have a predictive value with regard to fetal outcome (Kühnert et al, 1998a). Additionally, it was found that fetal pulse oximetry is capable of predicting developing acidosis by determining the duration of hypoxemia as indicated by an $FSpO_2$ of less than 30%. A decline of 0.002 pH units per 10 minutes was seen when the $FSpO_2$ was between 30% and 60%. A more rapid decline in pH (0.02 per 10 minutes) was observed when the $FSpO_2$ was less than 30%. When the $FSpO_2$ was less than 30% for more than 15 minutes, pH decreased in all cases. The pH dropped more rapidly when the $FSpO_2$ was continuously far below the 30% level. This research indicates that oxidative metabolism is in jeopardy when the fetal oxygen saturation remains lower than 30% for 10 minutes or more because of a progressive fall in pH (Seelbach-Göebel et al, 1999). $FSpO_2$, however, is not a measure of fetal arterial pH. In addition, fetal oxygen saturation can be more predictive of fetal status than scalp sampling for fetal pH because of the various factors such as caput formation and venous stasis that can influence pH values during the intrapartum/predelivery period.

U.S. randomized clinical trial on fetal pulse oximetry

In May 2000, the U.S. Food and Drug Administration approved the Nellcor fetal pulse oximetry technology (the OxiFirst Fetal Pulse Oximetry system including the N-400 monitor and fetal sensor) following a 3-year multicenter randomized clinical trial. The study was conducted concurrently in nine centers across the United States and was designed to test these hypotheses (Garite et al, 2000):

- The addition of fetal pulse oximetry to traditional electronic fetal monitoring will result in a clinically meaningful reduction of cesarean deliveries for the indication of nonreassuring fetal status.
- The addition of fetal pulse oximetry to traditional electronic fetal monitoring will permit the safe continuation of labor in the presence of a nonreassuring fetal heart rate pattern when the $FSpO_2$ is greater than or equal to 30% between contractions.
- The fetal sensor is safe for mother and fetus.

  The results of the study are as follows:

1. The study confirmed the primary hypothesis that the addition of fetal pulse oximetry to conventional electronic fetal monitoring reduced the rate of cesarean delivery for nonreassuring fetal status by more than 50%.
2. Fetal pulse oximetry significantly improved the sensitivity and specificity of surgical intervention for nonreassuring fetal status.
3. The use of a fetal pulse oximeter, a device that actually measures the parameter (fetal oxygenation) about which the clinician is concerned, allows more precise prediction and intervention for a more appropriate diagnosis (performing a cesarean delivery for the right indication at the right time). This has the potential to result in improved patient care.
4. The addition of fetal pulse oximetry had the unexpected benefit of improving the sensitivity of electronic fetal monitoring alone.
5. The continuation of labor in the presence of a nonreassuring FHR (with a reassuring $FSpO_2$) and a reduction in cesarean deliveries for nonreassuring fetal status, did not result in an apparent increase in adverse neonatal outcome.

6. The overall cesarean delivery rate remained unchanged because the rate of cesarean delivery for the single indication of dystocia was higher in the test group.

A follow-up study to address the sixth finding, an increase in the cesarean delivery rate for the indication of dystocia, was recently completed. The study concluded that cesarean delivery for dystocia is predictable in nulliparous women with normally oxygenated fetuses (FSpO$_2$ consistently >30) in the presence of significant nonreassuring FHR patterns (Porreco et al, 2003). This supports the indication of dystocia for cesarean delivery rather than nonreassuring fetal status because the fetus is well oxygenated. In addition, preparation time for a cesarean delivery in a controlled setting is possible because of reassuring pulse oximetry values.

Interpretation and management

A written clinical management protocol and procedure utilizing research-based findings of the RCT, subsequent clinical experience, and the manufacturer's clinical use guide should be in place in each institution using fetal pulse oximetry technology. The general guidelines for interpretation and management that follow are based on information from the U.S. randomized clinical trials on fetal pulse oximetry and more than 3 years of clinical experience following FDA approval of the technology (Garite et al, 2000; Swedlow, Bolling, 2003).

An FSpO$_2$ value greater than or equal to 30% between contractions is considered reassuring, and labor is generally allowed to continue unless otherwise indicated by the physician. If the value is less than 30% between contractions, or if fetal pulse oximetry information is not available, efforts to regain data (e.g., sensor adjustment, repositioning) should be made. However, if data are not present after readjustment, inferences regarding fetal status should not be made on the basis of earlier pulse oximetry values, and clinical management should be based on available data, such as the FHR pattern. Fetal pulse oximetry is an instantaneous measure of fetal oxygenation and is valid only at the time of measurement. If the pulse oximetry value is nonreassuring, conventional interventions aimed at improving the nonreassuring FHR patterns should be implemented while continuing to observe the pattern. The interventions include maternal position change, correction of maternal hypotension, improvement of maternal hydration, reduction or discontinuance of oxytocic drugs, and administration of supplemental oxygen (10 L/min by facemask). Other therapies include amnioinfusion to alleviate cord compression and the administration of tocolytic medication if the reduction of uterine activity is necessary. If the fetal oxygen saturation remains below 30% between contractions with a nonreassuring FHR pattern (class II in Table 6-2), evaluate and manage according to the available clinical data. Consideration of delivery by the most expeditious route may be warranted. If delivery is deemed necessary, the choice of delivery technique should be based on the condition of the woman and the fetus, the stage of labor, the pressure of time, and the skill of the provider (Kühnert et al, 1998b).

Fetal pulse oximetry is a promising new method of fetal assessment. Reduction in the cesarean delivery rate for the indication of nonreassuring fetal status by more than 50% was demonstrated through a rigorous, well-conducted multicenter clinical trial (Eglinton, Wolfson, 2000). The contribution of better methods of fetal assessment to decrease unnecessary interventions will be a major improvement in the provision of quality perinatal care (Simpson, 1998).

Umbilical Cord Acid–Base Determination

A useful adjunct to the Apgar score in assessing the immediate condition of the newborn is to obtain a sample of cord blood. Acid–base analysis of umbilical cord blood provides a more objective method of evaluating a newborn's condition than the Apgar score (ACOG, 1995b). Asphyxia, defined as hypercarbia, hypoxemia, and metabolic acidemia, is not measured by the Apgar score. Umbilical cord gas measurements reflect the oxygenation and acid–base status of the newborn at the time of delivery as well as the functioning of the placenta.

Indications for obtaining umbilical cord blood gases include the following:
- Nonreassuring fetal heart rate patterns
- Preterm delivery
- Emergency cesarean delivery
- Presence of maternal or fetal risk factors
- Assisted delivery with forceps or vacuum
- Thick meconium
- Low Apgar scores reflecting CNS depression
  There are no contraindications to obtaining cord gases.

Fetal condition is reflected by umbilical *artery* cord gas, whereas placental function is reflected by the umbilical *vein* cord gas. Normal findings preclude the presence of acidemia at or immediately before delivery (Gregg, Weiner, 1993).

Normal values for cord blood are summarized in the following chart (ACOG, 1995b; Helwig, 1996; Parer, 1997):

Normal values for cord blood

Cord Blood	pH	P_{CO_2} (mm Hg)	P_{O_2} (mm Hg)	Bicarbonate (meq/L)	Base Deficit (mmol/L)
Arterial (range)	7.27 (7.15-7.42)	49 (31.1-74.3)	17 (3.8-33.8)	22.3 (13.3-27.5)	0-11
Venous (range)	7.35 (7.24-7.49)	40.0 (23.2-49.2)	29.0 (15.4-48.2)	20.4 (15.0-24.7)	0-11

Base deficit is the numerical value expressed when the amount of bicarbonate in the blood gas is less than normal. Base excess is the numerical value expressed when the amount of bicarbonate in the blood gas is greater than normal. A neonate is considered to be acidemic if the blood gas pH is 7.10 to 7.18. Respiratory acidosis, in which the P_{CO_2} is increased and the bicarbonate is normal, is associated with an acute insult that is short in duration. Neonates born with evidence of metabolic acidosis have a normal P_{CO_2} level but a decrease in the amount of bicarbonate. Mixed acidosis is evidenced by an elevated P_{CO_2} level and a decrease in the amount of bicarbonate. With either metabolic or mixed acidosis, the fetus has had a longer and more profound insult for which it has not been able to compensate. The *type of acidosis (respiratory, metabolic, or mixed)* is based on the deviation from normal blood gas values, as shown in the following chart.

Types of acidosis

Blood Gases	Respiratory	Metabolic	Mixed
pH	↓	↓	↓
P_{CO_2}	↑	Normal	↑
HCO_3^-	Normal	↓	↓
Base deficit	Normal	↑	↑

Identification of fetal acid–base status is used to provide a basis for clinical management. The following rapid acid–base analysis tool is used by some facilities to quickly analyze cord blood gas:

- If the *arterial* pH is <7.10, it is acidosis.
- Look at the *base deficit.* This helps determine the type of acidosis.
    - If base deficit is *normal,* look at the P_{CO_2}. If it is >60, it is *respiratory* acidosis.
    - If the base deficit is >12 and the P_{CO_2} is normal (<60), it is *metabolic* acidosis.
    - If the base deficit is >12 and the P_{CO_2} is elevated (>60), it is *mixed* acidosis.

The procedure for obtaining umbilical cord blood consists of double-clamping a 10- to 20-cm (approximately 4- to 8-inch) segment of the umbilical cord immediately after delivery of the infant. A specimen should be drawn with a 1-ml plastic syringe that has been flushed with heparin solution (1000 U/ml). Draw blood from the umbilical artery first, then from the umbilical vein. Separate syringes should be used if drawing blood from both the umbilical vein and the umbilical artery.

Interventions for Nonreassuring Fetal Status

Amnioinfusion

Amnioinfusion is a useful technique to alleviate variable decelerations unresponsive to conventional therapies. The procedure involves administering room temperature normal saline or Ringer's lactate solution via the double-lumen intrauterine pressure catheter by either a gravity flow or an infusion pump. It significantly resolves moderate to severe variable decelerations by providing a cushion for the umbilical cord, and it provides a prophylactic approach to treat documented oligohydramnios either from a premature rupture of membranes or from decreasing placental function. It may also be very effective in diluting thick meconium-stained amniotic fluid. It is *not* a therapy to treat decreased variability or late decelerations (Miyazaki, Nevarez, 1985; Simpson, Creehan, 2001).

An amnioinfusion generally begins by administering a bolus of fluid (250 to 500 ml) over 20 to 30 minutes. The maintenance dose is infused at a rate of 2 to 3 ml/min (maximum of 180 ml/hr), during which time it is imperative that the amount of fluid returning is approximated and documented to avoid overdistention of the uterus. Assessment of the output can be accomplished by weighing the absorbent pads underneath the woman (1 ml = 1 gram) and counting the number of pads changed. Assessment of uterine resting tone is also an important aspect of surveillance during the procedure, and it should not exceed 40 mm Hg. It is unlikely that more than 1000 ml of fluid need be administered, and if variable decelerations persist even after this amount of fluid has been instilled into the uterus, other therapies should be used as treatment. Iatrogenic polyhydramnios may cause a placental abruption or pressure on the maternal diaphragm causing shortness of breath, tachycardia, and a change in maternal blood pressure. A rapid release or "gush" of fluid predisposes the woman to a prolapsed umbilical cord. The preterm fetus may benefit from a warmed solution, thus avoiding bradycardia. A blood warmer is the safest method for administering warmed fluid; fluid warmed in a microwave or blanket warmer should *not* be used for this purpose (Simpson, Creehan, 2001). Warmed fluid is also suggested if the rate of the amnioinfusion exceeds 15 ml/min.

There are a variety of ways to perform an amnioinfusion. It is important that the institution has a policy and procedure in place and that these are followed.

Indications for amnioinfusion

1. Laboring preterm women with premature rupture of the membranes (prophylactic)
2. Variable decelerations uncorrectable with conventional interventions
3. Significant oligohydramnios (amniotic fluid index ≤5) at term when labor is being induced
4. Presence of moderate to thick ("pea soup") meconium (Box 6-1)

Equipment and supplies

- Normal saline or Ringer's lactate solution, 1000 ml at room temperature
- Intrauterine catheter equipment, preferably with a double lumen and amnioport (if using single-lumen water-filled intrauterine pressure catheter, IV extension tubing with twin sites or arterial line [12 inches] and a three-way stopcock are needed)

Box 6-1   Meconium

Intrauterine passage of meconium can occur as a result of a hypoxic insult, but it can also occur in the absence of hypoxia. The density and concentration of meconium are a reflection of the amount of amniotic fluid. Thick meconium reflects some degree of oligohydramnios (Garite, 2002). Intrapartum amnioinfusion for meconium-stained fluid significantly improves neonatal outcome, lowers the cesarean delivery rate, and does not increase the postpartum endometritis rate (Pierce et al, 2000).

- Volumetric infusion pump and tubing, or IV pole for gravity flow
- Blood warmer or blood/fluid warming set (optional)

Procedure

Amnioinfusion should be initiated after insertion of the intrauterine catheter. Before the procedure, the intrauterine resting tone should be noted with the woman in the right and left lateral and supine positions for later comparison. Various procedures have been discussed in the literature, and each institution determines its own obstetrical policies and procedures. A sample procedure follows:

1. Connect the 1000-ml bottle of amnioinfusion solution to the IV tubing.
2. Flush the tubing with the solution.
3. Connect the tubing to the woman's intrauterine pressure catheter (IUPC) via the amnioport or double-lumen IUPC, or via a three-way stopcock, depending on the type of IUPC used.
4. Initiate the flow of amnioinfusion and instill the initial bolus, usually 250 to 500 ml over a 20- to 30-minute period (10 to 15 ml/min) using either an infusion pump or gravity flow. If gravity flow is used, the solution must be hung about 3 to 4 feet above the level of the tip of the IUPC. If fluid will not run by gravity, check the position/placement of the IUPC.
5. When variable decelerations resolve, continue the infusion at a slower rate, usually about 2 to 3 ml/min (120 to 180 ml/hr), as ordered by the care provider. If variable decelerations are not relieved after infusing 800 to 1000 ml of solution, the procedure is discontinued and alternative interventions are performed.

6. Observe and evaluate for amount and character of vaginal drainage. Vaginal output is assessed and documented to demonstrate that the volume infused is also coming back out and not causing overdistension of the uterus. Be vigilant for sudden "gushes" of fluid and assess for cord prolapse.

NOTE: Intrauterine resting tone will appear higher than normal, from 25 to 40 mm Hg, because of resistance to outflow through the tiny holes in the tip of the catheter. The true resting tone can be checked by temporarily discontinuing the flow of infusion.

Patient care

Care of the woman undergoing amnioinfusion includes the following:

1. Stop the infusion periodically, approximately every 30 to 60 minutes, to note the baseline uterine pressure. If the resting tone of the uterus exceeds 40 mm Hg, discontinue the infusion and notify the physician.
2. Change the underpads frequently to ensure the woman's comfort.
3. Note the color and amount of fluid on the underpads. The underpads may be weighed. Amounts of fluid returned should be determined (1 ml = 1 gram).
4. Monitor the woman for signs and symptoms of infection.
5. Monitor for signs and symptoms of cardiac or respiratory compromise secondary to an overexpanded uterus (maternal shortness of breath, hypotension, or tachycardia).
6. Monitor for resolving, concerning, or nonreassuring fetal heart rate patterns on the electronic fetal monitoring strip. Bradycardia may occur with cold or rapid infusion.
7. Once the reason for the procedure (e.g., variable decelerations, thick meconium-stained fluid) is resolved, the amnioinfusion may be discontinued.

Intrapartal Tocolysis Therapy for Nonreassuring FHR Patterns

Although tocolytic therapy is routinely used to prevent and manage preterm labor, it can be used as an adjunct to other interventions in the management of nonreassuring FHR patterns. When the fetus is not tolerating uterine activity and is not responsive to position change and discontinuance of the oxytocin infusion, an intravenous or subcutaneous injection of terbutaline can be administered while preparations are being made for immediate delivery. A cesarean delivery may be performed if the nonreassuring FHR pattern persists and the fetus cannot be safely delivered vaginally. On the other hand, if the FHR pattern improves, the woman may be allowed to continue labor. Terbutaline, which has a shorter time of onset, is generally preferred to magnesium sulfate, which has a longer time of onset. If the woman delivers shortly after the administration of a terbutaline or magnesium sulfate bolus, there is a risk of uterine atony and postpartum hemorrhage. Therefore appropriate preparations should be made if delivery appears imminent.

Nitroglycerin, a potent smooth muscle relaxant and vasodilator, has been used for acute tocolysis on selected women for indications such as shoulder dystocia, acute hypertonus with fetal distress, head entrapment of preterm infants, delivery of the head in difficult cesarean and breech deliveries, and persistent bradycardia during set-up for cesarean delivery. It has been administered by aerosol sublingual spray, by sublingual tablet, by transdermal patch, and intravenously. Nitroglycerin (glyceryl trinitrate) can cause hypotension and compensatory sympathetic responses leading to tachycardia; therefore it is used very selectively to effect uterine relaxation for acute tocolysis (Black et al, 1999).

Intrapartal tocolytic drugs

Any one of the following may be ordered by the physician to effect a reduction in uterine activity (Valenzuela, Foster, 1990; ACOG, 1995c; Brown, 1998):

- Terbutaline, 0.125 to 0.25 mg by slow IV push (1 minute)
- Terbutaline, 0.25 mg subcutaneously
- Magnesium sulfate, 2 g by slow IV push (1 minute)
- Magnesium sulfate, 4 g IV infusion over 20 minutes
- Nitroglycerin for acute intrapartal tocolysis per institutional protocol

References

American Academy of Pediatrics (AAP), American College of Obstetricians and Gynecologists (ACOG): *Guidelines for perinatal care,* ed 5, Washington, DC, 2002, The Academy and the College.

American College of Obstetricians and Gynecologists: Fetal heart rate patterns: Monitoring, interpretation, and management, *Technical Bulletin* No. 207, Washington, DC, July 1995a, The College.

American College of Obstetricians and Gynecologists: Umbilical artery blood acid–base analysis, *Technical Bulletin* no. 216, Washington, DC, Nov 1995b, The College.

American College of Obstetricians and Gynecologists: Preterm labor, *Technical Bulletin* no. 206, Washington, DC, Nov 1995c, The College.

American College of Obstetricians and Gynecologists: Inappropriate use of the terms fetal distress and birth asphyxia, *Committee Opinion* no. 197, Washington, DC, Feb 1998, The College.

American College of Obstetricians and Gynecologists, American Academy of Pediatrics: *Neonatal encephalopathy and cerebral palsy: Defining the pathogenesis and pathophysiology,* Washington, DC, 2003, The College and the Academy.

Association of Women's Health, Obstetric, and Neonatal Nurses*: Fetal heart monitoring: Principles and practices,* ed 3, Dubuque, Iowa, 2003, Kendall/Hunt.

Black RS, Lees C, Thompson C, et al: Maternal and fetal cardiovascular effects of transdermal glyceryl trinitrate and intravenous ritodrine, *Obstet Gynecol* 94(4):572-576, 1999.

Brown CE: Intrapartal tocolysis: An option for acute intrapartal fetal crisis, *J Obstet Gynecol Neonatal Nurs* 27(3):257-261, 1998.

Dicker D, Gingold A, Peleg D, et al: Effect of intracranial pressure changes on the fetal heart rate: Study of a hydrocephalic fetus, *Isr J Med Sci* 19(4):364-367, 1983.

Dildokar S, Mutch M: Major/multiple congenital anomalies and intrapartum fetal heart rate patterns, *South Dakota J Med* 33(9):5-9, 1979.

Dildy GA, Clark SL, Loucks CA: Intrapartum fetal pulse oximetry: Past, present, and future, *Am J Obstet Gynecol* 175(1):1-9, 1996.

Eglinton G, Wolfson R: Testimony at the 62nd meeting of the Obstetrics and Gynecology Panel of the FDA, Jan 24, 2000, p. 213; available at http://www.fda.gov/ohrms/dockets/ac/00/transcripts/3587t1.rtf.

Freeman RK, Garite TJ, Nageotte MP: *Fetal heart rate monitoring,* Baltimore, 2003, Williams & Wilkins.

Garite TJ: Intrapartum fetal evaluation. In Gabbe SG, Niebyl JR, Simpson JL, editors: *Obstetrics: Normal and problem pregnancies,* ed 4, New York, 2002, Churchill Livingstone.

Garite TJ, Dildy GA, McNamara H, et al: A multicenter controlled trial of fetal pulse oximetry in the intrapartum management of nonreassuring fetal heart rate patterns, *Am J Obstet Gynecol* 183(5):1049-1058, 2000.

Garite TJ, Porreco RP: Evaluating fetal hypoxia with pulse oximetry, *Contemp Ob Gyn* 46(7):12-26, 2001.

Goodwin TM, Milner-Masterson CL, Paul RH: Elimination of fetal scalp blood sampling on a large clinical service, *Obstet Gynecol* 83(6):971-974, 1994.

Gregg AR, Weiner CP: "Normal" umbilical arterial and venous acid–base and blood gas values, *Clin Obstet Gynecol* 35(1):24-32, 1993.

Hankins GDV: Apgar scores: Are they enough? *Contemp Ob Gyn (Ob-Gyn Law* special issue) 36:13-25, 1991.

Helwig IT, Parer JT, Kilpatrick SJ, Laros RK Jr: Umbilical cord blood acid–base state: What is normal? *Am J Obstet Gynecol* 174(6):1807-1814, 1996.

King T, Parer JT: The physiology of fetal heart rate patterns and perinatal asphyxia, *J Perinat Neonatal Nurs* 14(3):19-39, 2000.

Kühnert M, Seelbach-Göebel BS, Butterwegge M: Predictive agreement between the fetal arterial oxygen saturation and fetal scalp pH: Results of the German multicenter study, *Am J Obstet Gynecol* 178(2):330-335, 1998a.

Kühnert M, Seelbach-Göbel B, Di Renzo GC, et al: Guidelines for the use of fetal pulse oximetry during labor and delivery, *Perinat Neonatal Med* 3(4):432-433, 1998b.

MacLennan A: A template for defining a causal relationship between acute intrapartum events and cerebral palsy: International consensus statement, *BMJ* 319(7217):1054-1059, 1999.

Miyazaki FS, Nevarez F: Saline amnioinfusion for relief of repetitive variable decelerations: A prospective randomized study, *Am J Obstet Gynecol* 153(3):301-306, 1985.

National Institute of Child Health and Human Development Research Planning Workshop: Electronic fetal heart rate monitoring: Research guidelines for interpretation, *Am J Obstet Gynecol* 17(6):1385-1390, 1997.

Ombelet W, Van der Merwe JV: Sinusoidal fetal heart rate pattern associated with congenital hydrocephalus, *S Afr Med J* 67(11):423-425, 1985.

Parer JT: *Handbook of fetal heart rate monitoring,* Philadelphia, 1997, Saunders.

Pierce J, Gaudier FL, Sanchez-Ramos L: Intrapartum amnioinfusion for meconium-stained fluid: Meta-analysis of prospective clinical trials, *Obstet Gynecol* 95(6 Pt 2):1051-1056, 2000.

Porreco RP, Boehm F, Dildy G, et al: Dystocia in nulliparous patients monitored with fetal pulse oximetry, *Am J Obstet Gynecol* 187(6):S57, 2003.

Seelbach-Göebel B, Heupel M, Kühnert M, et al: The prediction of fetal acidosis by means of intrapartum pulse oximetry, *Am J Obstet Gynecol* 180(1):73-81; correction printed in *Am J Obstet Gynecol* 180(4):1048, 1999.

Simpson KR: Intrapartum fetal oxygen saturation monitoring, *Lifelines* 2(6):21-24, 1998.

Simpson KR, Creehan PA: *Perinatal nursing,* ed 2, Philadelphia, 2001, Lippincott.

Skupski DW, Rosenberg CR, Eglinton GS: Intrapartum fetal stimulation tests: A meta-analysis, *Obstet Gynecol* 99(1):129-134, 2002.

Swedlow DB: *Review of evidence for a fetal SpO₂ critical threshold of 30%,* Pleasanton, Calif, 1998, Nellcor.

Swedlow D, Bolling M: Personal communication. Letter to clinicians regarding changes in the management protocol for use of fetal pulse oximetry. (www.fda.gov/cdrh/psn/show16-Nellcor.html). (Nellcor, Pleasanton, Calif.), Feb. 3, 2003.

Valenzuela GJ, Foster T: Use of magnesium sulfate to treat hyperstimulation in term labor, *Obstet Gynecol* 75(5):762-764, 1990.

Van der Moer P, Gerretsen G, Visser GH: Fixed fetal heart rate pattern after intrauterine accidental decerebration, *Obstet Gynecol* 65(1): 125-127, 1985.

Influence of Gestational Age on Fetal Heart Rate Interpretation

Current guidelines for interpreting data from the electronic fetal monitor do not take into account prematurity and the developing fetus. Research has focused on monitoring as used for term or near-term gestations, but the characteristics and norms of the preterm fetus are different from those of the term fetus. Gestational age influences the baseline heart rate, the appearance and amplitude of accelerations, the fluctuations of variability, and the degree of development of cyclic fetal behavioral states. Monitoring of the smaller fetus and uterus may present significant challenges in both collection and interpretation of data. Clinicians must build a foundation on which to base their assessments when the fetus requires antenatal surveillance because of a fetal concern, maternal pathology, or a problem related to the pregnancy. An understanding of fetal physiology throughout the gestation is necessary for appropriate interpretation and intervention when the preterm (<35-week) fetus is monitored.

Furthermore, the postterm fetus has gestational-age-related characteristics different from those of the preterm and term fetus. Again, the physiological differences (e.g., in sleep and wake cycles) demonstrated by the fetus in the advanced gestational stage must be understood to interpret the fetal monitoring data.

This chapter will discuss the physiological characteristics of the preterm fetus and the postterm fetus and relate these characteristics to the interpretation of fetal monitoring data and assessment of fetal well-being.

Preterm Fetus

Heart rate patterns of preterm fetuses are different from those of full-term fetuses. The following are fetal heart rate characteristics of the preterm fetus.

- Average baseline rate is 150 to 155 beats per minute (bpm).
- Variability is not yet quantified by research.
- Accelerations are of lower amplitude (10 bpm × 10 sec) until 32 weeks.
- Episodic variable decelerations occur in a normal preterm fetus of 20 to 30 weeks.
- Periodic variable decelerations occur twice as often during the intrapartum period.
- Progression from reassuring to nonreassuring status is more rapid.
- Prior to 26 weeks, fetus is unresponsive to vibroacoustic stimulation (VAS).
- Between 20 and 30 weeks of gestation, *decelerations* are more commonly associated with fetal movement than accelerations.

Baseline Fetal Heart Rate in the Preterm Fetus

The fetal heart rate baseline rate decreases as gestational age increases. As discussed in Chapter 2, the sympathetic branch of the autonomic nervous system dominates responses until about 32 weeks of gestation, when the maturation of the parasympathetic branch results in parasympathetic domination. It is more likely that the preterm fetus will have a baseline rate on the higher side of normal (110 to 160 bpm), decreased variability, and decreased amplitude and number of accelerations without this being evidence of compromise. The tracing of the preterm fetus also demonstrates a limited number of pronounced changes in overall appearance related to rest and activity states (Eganhouse, Burnside, 1992).

Periodic and Episodic Heart Rate Changes in the Preterm Fetus

Accelerations of the fetal heart rate in association with fetal movement begin to occur late in the second trimester of pregnancy. Between 20 and 30 weeks, however, it is more common to see 12- to 20-second spontaneous *decelerations* of the fetal heart rate

(FHR) as a response to fetal activity (Pillai, James, 1990). Asystole may occur in week 22 to 24, and it appears as a signal loss on the tracing. This may be a vagal response or simply a reflection of the immaturity of both branches of the autonomic nervous system (Sorokin et al, 1982) (Figures 7-1 and 7-2).

Because fetal heart rate reactivity is a function of fetal maturity, more than 15% of nonstress tests performed before 32 weeks of gestation may be nonreactive without being indicative of fetal compromise (AAP, ACOG, 2002). Prior to 32 weeks, most fetuses do not demonstrate the accelerations of 15 beats × 15 seconds that are required for the tracing to be interpreted as reactive (Castillo, 1989; NICHD, 1997). At less than 32 weeks of gestation, an acceleration is defined as having an acme of 10 or more beats above the baseline with a duration of 10 seconds (NICHD, 1997).

After 32 weeks of gestation, appearances of reactivity increase dramatically. The synchronous cyclic fetal behavior reported by Johnson and colleagues (1988) and Pillai and James (1990) also

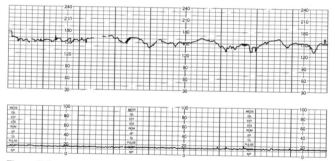

Figure 7-1

This woman was evaluated for complaints of cramping at 22 weeks of gestation. Baseline FHR is 155 bpm with low-amplitude accelerations. Variable decelerations of minimal depth and duration are often seen when the woman or provider is unable to discern uterine activity (Sorokin, 1982). FHR accelerations of 10 bpm for 10 seconds or more are more commonly seen in the fetus less than 32 weeks, but accelerations of 15 bpm for 15 seconds may be seen in this tracing. Once the fetus demonstrates this reactive criterion, it is expected to continue doing so when normoxic.

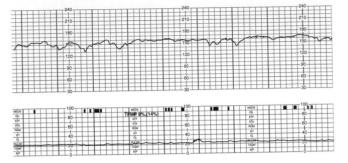

Figure 7-2
This 25-week fetus demonstrated mild variable decelerations
and a baseline of 160 bpm, both normal at this gestational
age. As the parasympathetic branch of the autonomic
nervous system develops, the baseline rate decreases and
the variability increases.

begins to appear at this gestational age (Figure 7-3). The following
are characteristic changes in the heart rate that occur with fetal
maturation.

- Decrease in baseline rate from upper limits toward lower limits
- Increase in the amplitude of variability (cyclic changes around
  the baseline)
- Increase in the extremes of variability between sleep and wake
  states
- Increase in both the number and the amplitude of accelerations
- Decrease in the time between accelerations
- Decrease in the number of decelerations

Because of the inconsistent relationship between accelerations
and fetal movement, the nonstress test is a poor guide to fetal
behavior and well-being prior to 28 weeks of gestation in many
fetuses. It is preferable to use a biophysical profile and ultrasound
visualization of fetal movement in the fetus less than 28 weeks.
Appropriate norms need to be established for the fetus that is less
than 32 weeks of gestation. Rather than using the terms *reactive* or
nonreactive, it would be more accurate to document findings as
appropriate for gestational age. Most important, once a fetus demonstrates a reactive nonstress test, any subsequent failure to do so must
register suspicion of compromise and requires further evaluation.

Behavior States in the Preterm Fetus

Fetuses predictably develop recognizable patterns of behavior or "states" as gestation progresses, and these are similar to states observed in the newborn. The changes in behavioral states occur in a coordinated pattern in the healthy fetus beginning at 35 weeks. Adequate uteroplacental function and fetal oxygenation are

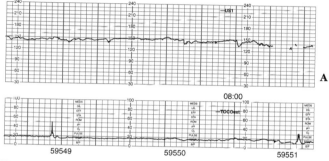

Figure 7-3
The cyclic behavior of the near-term fetus (gestational age, 35 weeks). A significant difference in both variability and the presence of accelerations correlates with sleep and wake states. **A,** 1F behavior is demonstrated with the quiet sleep state. Accelerations are absent and the variability is decreased.

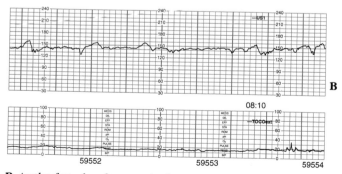

B, As the fetus has frequent body movements during active sleep (2F), accelerations are evidenced and the variability increases to become moderate.

Continued

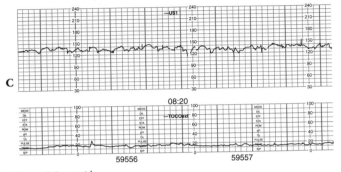

Figure 7-3, cont'd

C, In the quiet awake state (3F), moderate variability continues with only occasional accelerations.

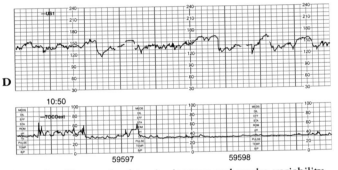

D, In the 4F state, the fetus is vigorous and awake, variability increases, and accelerations merge and coalesce.

necessary for the fetus to accomplish and maintain these healthy patterns of behavior. Whereas infant states are determined by characteristics of cardiac and respiratory regulation, eyes open or closed, motor activity, and the presence of rapid eye movements (REM) during sleep, fetal states are recognized by the regulation of the fetal heart rate, the presence of eye movements, and fetal activity. Sleep changes develop with maturation of the central nervous system (CNS) (Blackburn, 2003). Four behavioral states have been identified and verified by real-time ultrasound (Table 7-1). The maturing fetus shifts from one behavioral state to another in a coordinated cyclic manner. Pronounced fetal heart rate variations and changes occur with both sleep and wake cycles. The preterm

Table 7-1   Fetal behavioral states

State	Behavior	Associated FHR Pattern
1F: Quiet sleep	Absence of rapid eye movement (REM); infrequent body and startle movements; rhythmic mouthing movements	Regular/stable fetal heart rate; minimal variability; rare accelerations with fetal movement (FM)
2F: Active sleep	Frequent body movements; abrupt head and limb movement; REM	Minimal to moderate variability; frequent accelerations with FM
3F: Quiet awake	Infrequent body movements, REM	Moderate variability
4F: Active awake	Continuous and vigorous movement	Moderate to marked variability; frequent accelerations fusing into tachycardia

From Blackburn ST: *Maternal, fetal, and neonatal physiology: A clinical perspective,* ed 2, St. Louis, 2003, Saunders; Druzin ML, Gabbe SG, Reed KL: Antepartum fetal evaluation. In Gabbe SG, Niebyl JR, Simpson JL, editors: *Obstetrics: Normal and problem pregnancies,* ed 4, New York, 2002, Churchill Livingstone; Harman CR, Menticoglou S, Manning FA: Assessing fetal health. In James DK, Steer PJ, Weiner CP, Gonik B, editors: *High risk pregnancy: Management options,* ed 2, Philadelphia, 1999, Bailliere Tindall; Richardson BS, Gagnon R: Fetal breathing and body movements. In Creasy RK, Resnik R: *Maternal-fetal medicine,* ed 4, Philadelphia, 1999, Saunders.

fetus spends the majority of time in the quiet sleep state (1F), whereas the term fetus spends most of the time in the active sleep state (2F). As gestation advances closer to term, the fetus remains in any particular state for approximately 20 to 40 minutes (Johnson et al, 1988).

Asynchronous cycles between rest and activity have been reported at as early as 31 weeks of gestation. These behavioral states must be considered when interpreting the fetal heart rate patterns. For example, misinterpretations can occur when there is a change in the baseline rate during the active awake 4F state or when there is a possible hypoxemic tracing with a lack of accelerations and decreased variability during 1F. The differences in baseline variability associated with the active and the quiet states become much more apparent as gestation advances to the 36th week (Figure 7-4).

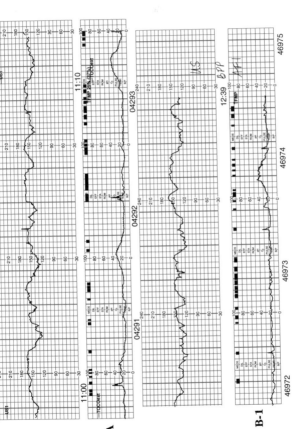

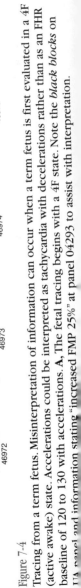

Figure 7-4

Tracing from a term fetus. Misinterpretation of information can occur when a term fetus is first evaluated in a 4F (active awake) state. Accelerations could be interpreted as tachycardia with decelerations rather than as an FHR baseline of 120 to 130 with accelerations. A, The fetal tracing begins with a 4F state. Note the *black blocks* on UA panel and information stating "increased FMP 25%" at panel 04293 to assist with interpretation.

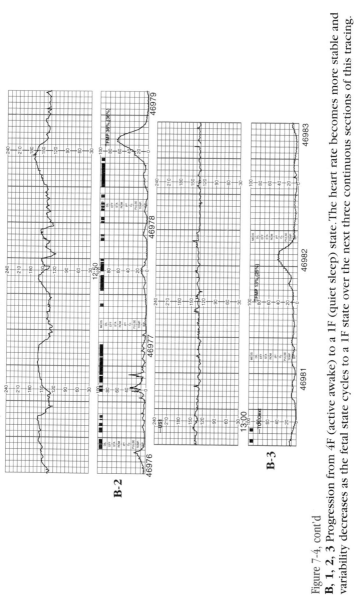

Figure 7-4, cont'd
B, 1, 2, 3 Progression from 4F (active awake) to a 1F (quiet sleep) state. The heart rate becomes more stable and variability decreases as the fetal state cycles to a 1F state over the next three continuous sections of this tracing.

Fetal Breathing Movements

Fetal breathing movements (FBM) occur in isolated bursts prior to the 24th week of gestation. These movements reflect CNS reactivity and response to metabolic and sensory stimuli. FBM contribute to lung fluid regulation and lung growth in the fetus. The movement of the diaphragm is needed for development of chest wall muscle and the diaphragm, providing strength for the initial breath at birth (Blackburn, 2003). As the fetus matures, FBM become periodic and regular in frequency and uniformity. Prior to 32 weeks, the breathing movements resemble panting. Between 24 and 26 weeks, FBM increase along with the number of gross body movements. After 32 weeks, the breathing movements are irregular with multiple inspiratory movements and prolonged expiratory phases. FBM noted on ultrasound increase in frequency and duration as gestation advances. A few days prior to the onset of term labor, breathing movements decrease. In advanced labor, they are rarely seen. A less dramatic reduction in FBM is observed when women are in preterm labor (Lowe, Reiss, 1996).

Fetal breathing movements require energy and adequate fetal oxygenation. A decrease in breathing motion in response to hypoxemia may be a protective measure to decrease oxygen consumption. Alterations in maternal and fetal carbon dioxide partial pressure (PCO_2) affect FBM. Increasing maternal PCO_2 increases FBM, whereas maternal hyperventilation decreases them (Lowe, Reiss, 1996). This is commonly reflected by repetitive variable decelerations, a fetal heart rate pattern suggestive of respiratory acidosis. An accompanying rise in the baseline rate and a loss of variability also indicate an increased fetal need for oxygen. The following are characteristics of fetal breathing movements:

- Associated with REM
- Associated with decreased FHR, increased variability, irregular oscillatory pattern
- Usually not associated with fetal activity but with fetal sleep
- Episodic and paradoxical
- Observed more frequently with advancing gestation, so that by the third trimester they can be observed 30% of the time
- Increased with glucose infusion, smoking, after meals
- Decreased with hypoxemia, alcohol ingestion, asphyxia, general anesthesia

- Decreased with labor (preterm as well as term)
- Increased from 7:00 P.M. to midnight, and decreased from 1:00 A.M. to 7:00 A.M.

Preterm Uterine Activity

Preterm uterine activity monitoring is technically challenging at less than 35 weeks of gestation. The smaller uterus may not accommodate effective placement of both toco and ultrasound transducers. Electronic fetal monitors used in hospitals may not be sensitive enough to detect and record preterm uterine activity, so it may be better to use palpation, alone or in combination with the electronic monitoring to confirm findings. Correct placement of the toco improves the accuracy of uterine activity assessment. Rather than placing the toco in the area of the fundus, positioning it below the umbilicus in an early (28-week) pregnancy will result in a more accurate assessment.

Low-Amplitude, High-Frequency Contractions

Complaints of cramping are often evaluated and termed either low-amplitude, high-frequency (LAHF) uterine contractions or irritability. LAHF contractions may be precursors to preterm labor contractions; these are often painless, but they require attention and further assessment (Figure 7-5). LAHF contractions may also be indicative of a placental abruption. A nonreassuring FHR in tandem with waves of cramping or irritability may be indicative of an abruption, and this needs further assessment and intervention. It is important to obtain a careful history and provide close observation of the FHR response.

All pregnant women should be well informed of the signs and symptoms of preterm labor and evaluated appropriately when they have complaints of any combination of these signs and symptoms. Preterm birth complicates 10% to 12% of all pregnancies (Freda, Patterson, 2001).

Painful uterine contractions in a pregnancy at low risk for preterm delivery make accurate diagnosis difficult. Because preterm delivery accounts for 80% of fetal morbidity and mortality, health care providers often exercise caution and administer tocolytic medications even when there has been no cervical change or other evidence of true preterm labor.

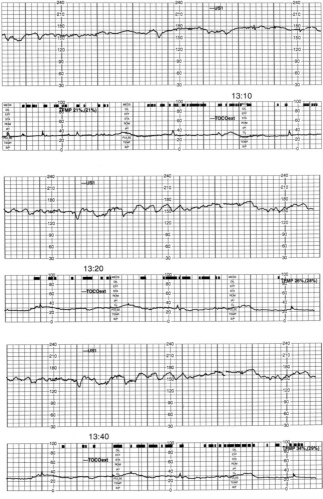

Figure 7-5
At 32 weeks of gestation, this woman with a history of a preterm delivery is evaluated for cramping. Low-amplitude, high-frequency (LAHF) contractions are noted.

Tocolytic Agents and Effect on FHR

Most tocolytic protocols are planned to minimize the occurrence of maternal side effects. In contrast, the protocols for administering indomethacin (Indocin), a prostaglandin synthetase inhibitor, are planned to protect the fetus from potentially life-threatening morbidities (e.g., constriction of the ductus arterious and a decrease in renal function resulting in a decrease in amniotic fluid). Therapy is often limited to 48 hours and to gestations of less than 32 weeks. Assessment of amniotic fluid volume is performed at the initiation of therapy and whenever a decision is made to prolong indomethacin therapy. Prolonged therapy is usually accompanied by daily ultrasonography to evaluate for developing oligohydramnios and evaluation of the fetal ductus arteriosus. It is necessary to observe the fetal heart rate pattern for variable decelerations signifying umbilical cord compression, which is seen more commonly with a decrease in amniotic fluid volume (Rodts-Palenik, Morrison, 2002).

The calcium-channel blocker *nifedipine* (Procardia) may cause a mild increase in maternal heart rate and a modest decrease in diastolic blood pressure. This may cause diminished uterine blood flow, resulting in fetal hypoxemia manifesting as late decelerations, a rise in baseline FHR, or, if not corrected, a decrease in variability (Rodts-Palenik, Morrison, 2002).

The beta-sympathomimetic *terbutaline* (Brethine) causes maternal tachycardia and an increase in oxygen consumption. Fetal tachycardia often parallels maternal tachycardia and may lead to decreasing variability. With prolonged use of the beta-mimetic, fetal arrhythmia may develop as well.

Magnesium sulfate, the most commonly used medication for tocolysis, has been associated with decreases of both baseline variability and accelerations. However, there is no conclusive research evidence that this is true. In a small study, Heitt and colleagues (1995) report a decrease in the amplitude of accelerations and in variability with a magnesium level of greater than 4.6 mEq/L. Other studies have found no relationship between magnesium sulfate administration and changes in fetal heart rate variability. When a decrease in variability and a loss of accelerations are observed during the administration of magnesium sulfate, it is important to use the fetal values prior to medication administration as the control and then assess baseline rate, presence of accelerations, and absence of decelerations after treatment. Utilizing the

Figure 7-6

Tracing of primigravida at 27 weeks' gestation with a history of preterm premature rupture of membranes. There is commonly a rapid progression from reassuring to nonreassuring fetal status in the preterm fetus. The combination of the change in variability and variable decelerations often leads to lower Apgar scores and lower cord gases. **A,** Admission tracing of an afebrile woman, who is placed on antibiotics. **B,** The woman is monitored on day 6 of hospitalization. She has a fever of 102° F and is prescribed an additional antibiotic.

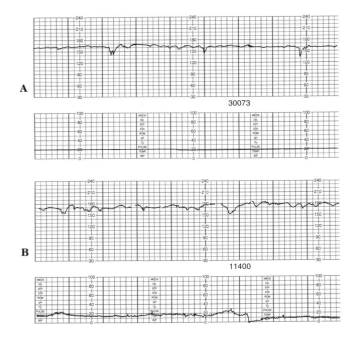

biophysical profile may provide a more complete evaluation of the fetal status in this situation.

The woman who presents in labor with a preterm fetus and premature rupture of membranes has an increased risk of developing a nonreassuring fetal heart rate pattern. Her risk is far greater than that of the woman in preterm labor with intact membranes. Acute inflammatory changes are associated with an intra-amniotic infection

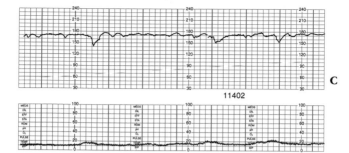

Figure 7-6, cont'd
C, Note the FHR baseline of 170 bpm with variable decelerations.

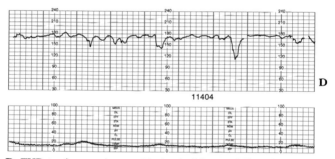

D, FHR tracing continues with the decision to deliver. Note increasing variable decelerations in addition to fetal tachycardia with a change in variability.

resulting in variable decelerations and decreasing variability when the gestation is less than 32 weeks (Salafia et al, 1998) (Figure 7-6).

The Postterm Fetus

The definition of *postterm pregnancy* has remained constant over several decades. It signifies a gestation of more than 42 weeks, or 294 days from the last menstrual period or 280 days from the conception date (Resnik, Caler, 1999; Spellacy, 1999). The incidence of postterm pregnancies is about 10%, but they account for a mortality of 2% to 4%, which is double that of the term fetus

(Divon, 2002). Pregnancy between 40 and 42 weeks of gestation may be termed *prolonged pregnancy*. *Postmature* describes the infant with recognized clinical features indicative of a postterm fetus. The term *postdates* has been abandoned as a description of the fetus who is older than 42 weeks of gestation (Spellacy, 1999).

Placental Function

Placental function peaks at 37 weeks of gestation when the placental surface area is greatest. If placental function remains *adequate,* the consequence of the postterm gestation may be macrosomia, leading to an increased risk of prolonged labor, shoulder dystocia, and birth trauma. If placental function *degenerates,* consequences are inadequate nutrition, a decrease in amniotic fluid, intrauterine growth restriction (IUGR), inadequate fetal oxygenation, and nonreassuring fetal heart rate patterns. The nonreassuring fetal heart rate patterns are a result of umbilical vessel compression from oligohydramnios, manifesting in the increased occurrence of variable decelerations. When nutritional deprivation progresses to decreased fetal oxygenation, late decelerations appear. A fetus that continues to be hypoxemic will not exhibit the usual interaction of the parasympathetic and sympathetic branches of the autonomic nervous system, and variability will be decreased. The need for more oxygen causes the fetus to increase its heart rate to obtain more oxygen, and tachycardia may result. The vagal response that follows compression of the umbilical cord may also increase the risk of meconium release. The function of the placenta may be adequate or inadequate as it matures or ages in the postterm fetus. *Adequate* placental function in the postterm fetus may be associated with the following factors:

- Macrosomia
- Prolonged labor
- Shoulder dystocia
- Dystocia or abnormal labor pattern
- Birth trauma

In contrast, when placental function is *inadequate* in the postterm fetus, it may be associated with the following:

- Inadequate nutrition: IUGR
- Oligohydramnios
- Cord compression, with resulting variable decelerations
- Hypoxemia: late decelerations, tachycardia, decreased variability
- Meconium passage

Baseline FHR of the Postterm Fetus

The baseline heart rate of the postterm fetus may be less than 110 bpm because of the maturity and dominance of the parasympathetic nervous system with its deceleratory influence and effect. The variability may be increased because of central nervous system maturity. A large discrepancy exists in the variability, which can be visualized in the awake (moderate to marked) versus fetal sleep (minimal) states of behavior.

Periodic and Episodic Changes in the Postterm Fetus

Autonomic nervous system development continues with advancing gestation, and periods of wakefulness and activity increase. Accelerations coalesce and may appear to be a change in baseline in the tachycardic range. Fetal heart rate patterns may mimic non-reassuring tracings or compromise when the fetus is sleeping (1F) or when the fetus is in the active awake (4F) state when pronounced and prolonged accelerations are noted (Figure 7-7).

The postterm pregnancy is associated with a decrease in both amniotic fluid and placental function. Continuous fetal monitoring may be helpful in early identification of nonreassuring FHR patterns. Assess the fetal tracing for these variations of the FHR:

- Variable decelerations as a result of oligohydramnios
- Late decelerations as a result of uteroplacental insufficiency
- Tachycardia, decreased accelerations, or decreased variability occurring as a result of hypoxemia

Behavioral States of the Postterm Fetus

The fetal heart rate is affected by behavioral states in the postterm fetus. For example, large variations in baseline variability and periodic or episodic changes may be visualized between sleep and awake cycles. The following characteristic FHR patterns related to behavioral states are observed in the postterm fetus:

1. FHR pattern may mimic nonreassuring patterns.
   - In the 4F state (active awake, vigorous activity), FHR may easily be misinterpreted as tachycardia with decelerations as accelerations become more prolonged with short returns to the baseline.
   - Decreased variability and absent accelerations in a healthy postterm fetus during labor are likely to represent sleep and not hypoxemia or compromise.

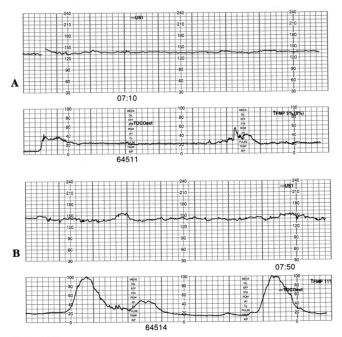

Figure 7-7

This 42-week fetus presents to the labor and delivery unit in a
sleep state (1F). **A,** The tracing represents the idea of "the
older the fetus, the flatter the tracing." **B,** A change in the
active sleep state (2F) is evidenced by accelerations
associated with frequent fetal body movements.

> NOTE: If decreased variability lasts longer than 40 minutes
> or the baseline rate rises, there may be a concern with
> oxygenation.

- In the 1F state (quiet sleep), the FHR pattern is unaffected by
  even the strongest uterine contractions of late labor.
- The older the fetus, the flatter is the tracing during the sleep
  cycles of 1F and 3F.

2. Pronounced and prolonged FHR accelerations are related to
   continuing development of autonomic nervous system with
   increased periods of wakefulness (4F state).

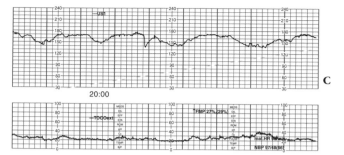

Figure 7-7, cont'd
C, In a coordinated pattern of behavior, the fetus enters the active wake state (4F) and merging accelerations are seen, associated with vigorous fetal activity.

NOTE: Accelerations of FHR in the postterm fetus are reassuring regardless of how the accelerations are elicited. In addition, a reactive nonstress test is highly reliable and reassuring. A nonreactive nonstress test is less reliable, and additional testing or a full biophysical profile may be beneficial.

Meconium

Meconium is not an independent sign of fetal compromise but rather an *outcome* of an event that may predispose to or be a consequence of fetal compromise. The pathophysiology of meconium release is a result of several factors:

- Normal gut function related to fetal maturity
- Hyperperistalsis and anal sphincter release in response to hypoxemia
- Vagal response to cord compression in the absence of hypoxemia
- A combination of these three factors

Ten to fifteen percent of live births occur in the presence of meconium, and in 35% of those newborns, the meconium is below the vocal cords (Rosenberg, 2002). Because the prevention of meconium aspiration is an important goal, it may be treated by the use of amnioinfusion (discussed in Chapter 6). In the presence of oligohydramnios, meconium fluid, and cord compression, aspiration of meconium-stained amnionitic fluid may occur as a result of hypoxemia, which may stimulate fetal gasping. Amnioinfusion is postulated to have a positive effect on neonatal outcome (Weismiller, 1998). Diluting thick meconium in the amniotic fluid may reduce the risk of meconium aspiration syndrome. It is most probably not the dilution of the meconium but the cushioning of the umbilical cord and the treatment (or prevention) of variable decelerations that diminishes the fetal gasping reflex.

Implications for Clinical Practice

Accurate fetal assessment and interpretation of fetal monitoring data depend on an understanding of changes in fetal physiology and fetal individuality throughout gestation. Characteristics of the preterm and postterm fetus must be considered alongside other clinical data. Whenever information is interpreted from electronic fetal monitoring and antepartum surveillance tests, fetal state or behavior must be considered along with gestational age. Be aware that meconium-stained fluid is not a reliable indicator of fetal compromise but rather a physiological event that occurs for a variety of reasons.

References

American Academy of Pediatrics (AAP), American College of Obstetricians and Gynecologists (ACOG): *Guidelines for perinatal care*, Washington, DC, 2002, The Academy and the College.

Baird S, Ruth D: Electronic fetal monitoring of the preterm fetus, *J Perinat Neonatal Nurs* 16(1):12-24, 2002.

Blackburn ST: *Maternal, fetal, and neonatal physiology: A clinical perspective*, ed 2, St Louis, 2003, Saunders.

Castillo R, Devoe LD, Arthur M, et al: The preterm non stress test: Effects of gestational age and length of study, *Am J Obstet Gynecol* 160(1): 172-175, 1989.

Divon MY: Prolonged pregnancy. In Gabbe S, Niebyl JR, Simpson JL, editors: *Obstetrics: Normal and problem pregnancies*, ed 4, New York, 2002, Churchill Livingstone.

Druzin ML, Gabbe SG, Reed KL: Antepartum fetal evaluation. In Gabbe SG, Niebyl JR, Simpson JL, editors: *Obstetrics: normal and problem pregnancies,* ed 4, New York, 2002, Churchill Livingstone.

Eganhouse D, Burnside S: Nursing assessment and responsibilities in monitoring the preterm pregnancy, *J Obstet Gynecol Neonatal Nurs* 21(5):355-363, 1992.

Freda MC, Patterson ET: *Preterm labor: Prevention and nursing management*, ed 2, White Plains, N.Y., 2001, March of Dimes.

Harman CR, Menticoglou S, Manning FA: Assessing fetal health. In James DK, Steer PJ, Weiner CP, Gonik B, editors: *High risk pregnancy: Management options,* ed 2, Philadelphia, 1999, Balliere Tindall.

Heitt AK, Devoe LD, Brown HI, Watson J: Effect of magnesium on fetal heart rate variability using computer analysis, *Am J Perinatol* 12(4): 259-261, 1995.

Johnson T, Besinger RE, Thomas RL, et al: New clues to fetal behavior and well being, *Contemp Ob Gyn* 31(5):108-123, 1988.

Lowe N, Reiss R: Parturition and fetal adaptation, *J Obstet Gynecol Neonatal Nurs* 25(4):339-349, 1996.

National Institute of Child Health and Human Development (NICHD) Research Planning Workshop: Electronic fetal heart rate monitoring: Research guidelines for interpretation, *Am J Obstet Gynecol* 17(6): 1385-1390, 1997.

Pillai M, James D: The development of fetal heart rate patterns during normal pregnancy, *Obstet Gynecol* 76(5):812-816, 1990.

Resnik R, Caler MD: Post-term pregnancy. In Creasy RK, Resnik R, editors: *Maternal-fetal medicine,* ed 4, Philadelphia, 1999, Saunders.

Richardson BS, Gagnon R: Fetal breathing and body movements. In Creasy RK, Resnik R, editors: *Maternal–fetal medicine,* ed 4, Philadelphia, 1999, Saunders.

Rodts-Palenik S, Morrison J: Tocolysis: An update for the practitioner, *Obstet Gynecol Surv* 57(5 suppl 2):S9-34, 2002.

Rosenberg AA: The neonate. In Gabbe S, Niebyl JR, Simpson JL, editors: *Obstetrics: Normal and problem pregnancies,* ed 4, New York, 2002, Churchill Livingstone.

Salafia CM, Ghidini A, Sherer DM, Pezzullo JC: Abnormalities of the fetal heart rate in preterm deliveries associate with acute intra-amniotic infection, *J Soc Gynecol Investig* 5(4):188-191, 1998.

Sorokin Y, Dierker LJ, Pillary SK, et al: The association between fetal heart patterns and fetal movements in pregnancies between 20 and 30 weeks gestation, *Am J Obstet Gynecol* 143(3):243-249, 1982.

Spellacy WN: Postdate pregnancy. In Scott JR, Hammond CB, Saia PJ, Spellacy WN, editors: *Danforth's obstetrics,* ed 8, Philadelphia, 1999, Lippincott Williams & Wilkins.

Weismiller D: Transcervical amnioinfusion, *Am Fam Physician* 57(3): 504-510, 1998.

Fetal Assessment in Non-Obstetrical Settings

8

Assessment and care of the pregnant woman takes place in a variety of settings. Collaboration among perinatal, perioperative, intensive care, and emergency department teams is essential when the pregnant woman is cared for in an area other than the labor and delivery suite. Knowledge of the physiological and anatomic adaptations of pregnancy is required because pregnancy alters anatomy and physiology to such an extent that clinical symptoms may be distorted and normal discomforts may contribute to a puzzling picture. Some changes are so dramatic that they would be considered pathological in the nonpregnant woman (Box 8-1). For example, palpation is difficult as the peritoneum stretches to allow displacement of the abdominal organs.

The laboratory values relied on for confirmation of a diagnosis or problem also differ, because of the adaptations required by the body during pregnancy. Furthermore, not only does the pregnant woman present with her unique challenges but she arrives with a *second* patient who also requires assessment, care, and possible intervention. Fetal stability depends on maternal stability. If caregivers do not support the adaptations of the pregnancy, there is a potential for adverse maternal and fetal events.

The focus of this chapter is to demonstrate the need for collaborative efforts when a pregnant woman requires evaluation. She needs the *right* providers to care for her at the *right* time and in the *right* setting. When she receives care outside of the perinatal unit, it is often because she requires surgical or medical expertise. The needs of the fetus should not be overlooked. The caregiver—the labor and delivery nurse or the nurse from the emergency department or critical care unit—must have the requisite skills and must be qualified to evaluate the fetus by education, experience, and

Box 8-1   Physiological Adaptations to Pregnancy

Cardiovascular

- Physiological anemia, hypervolemia (expansion of plasma volume greater than expansion of red cell mass)
- Blood volume increases by 30% to 40% (1200 to 1500 ml higher than prepregnant state)
- Plasma increases 70%, cells 30%
- Hematocrit of 32% to 34% is not unusual
- Cardiac output increases 30% to 50% (a result of increased blood volume)
- Heart rate and stroke volume increase
- Systemic vascular resistance decreases, with resultant decrease in blood pressure and mean arterial pressure
- Uteroplacental vascular bed is dilated; passive low resistance system
- Uterofetoplacental unit receives 20% of cardiac output
- Peripheral edema; dyspnea; presence of third heart sound
- Pelvic venous congestion

Hematological

- Increased clotting factors VII, VIII, IX, and X, and fibrinogen (hypercoagulable)
- Decreased serum albumin may lower colloid osmotic pressure (predisposing to pulmonary edema)

Renal

- Renal system receives 20% of cardiac output
- Glomerular filtration rate increase by 50%
- Increase in urinary stasis; susceptibility to urinary tract infections increases

Respiratory

- Tidal volume increases by 30% to 40%; respiratory rate unchanged
- Oxygen consumption increases by 20%

Continued

> ## Box 8-1   Physiological Adaptations to Pregnancy—cont'd
>
> - Diaphragm elevated by the growing fetus
> - Arterial P_{CO_2} decreases as a result of hyperventilation, resulting in a "compensated" respiratory alkalosis
>
> Gastrointestinal
>
> - Smooth muscle relaxes, increasing gastric emptying time
> - Gastric motility decreases, sphincters relax, higher likelihood of aspiration
> - Intestines pushed upward, relocating to the upper abdomen

performance standards. It is imperative that communication between services and providers be clear and timely to ensure that the maternal–fetal dyad receives appropriate care, regardless of the physical setting, by the most appropriate staff member.

Emergency Services Department Assessment and Care

Pregnant women present to the emergency department (ED) for a variety of reasons. A *primary* survey occurs at triage: "Why are you here?" A s*econdary* survey includes obtaining information about signs, symptoms, the mechanism of injury, and evaluation of pain. This is of course predicated on the woman's ability to communicate and the absence of trauma that would prevent communication.

Findings from the primary survey and identification of gestational age are usually the best indicators for the unit in which the woman's care would be most appropriately managed. Special attention to the pregnancy is a part of the assessment and not merely an afterthought. The pregnant woman must be viewed as two patients just as she would if she presented with her baby in her arms. Before discharge from the emergency department or transfer to another area, both patients require assessment to confirm maternal *and* fetal well-being. *Where* the assessment takes place is not the concern. Rather, it is *who* is performing the assessment and whether they are qualified by virtue of education and competency in obstetrics.

Women present to an emergency unit for numerous nonpregnancy and pregnancy-related reasons. Many emergency units use 20 weeks of gestation as a determinant of whether care should be managed in the ED or in labor and delivery. Women who present to the ED at a gestation of more than 20 weeks complaining of well-recognized obstetrical concerns (e.g., vaginal bleeding, contractions, rupture of membranes, increased or watery vaginal discharge, abdominal pain, pelvic pressure, decreased fetal movement) may be transferred immediately to the labor and delivery unit for further assessment and management. For those women with vague symptoms such as headache, edema, nausea and vomiting, or "just not feeling well," the decision about where to evaluate is not always so clear. These vague symptoms may be associated with the hypertensive disorders of pregnancy, such as pregnancy-induced hypertension or the HELLP syndrome (a severe form of preeclampsia characterized by hemolysis [H], elevated liver [EL] enzymes, and low platelets [LP]). Well-meaning care in a non-obstetrical setting for the woman with a hypertensive disorder of pregnancy has the potential of being detrimental to both the woman and the fetus. Alternatively, these vague symptoms could reflect influenza, food poisoning, cholecystitis, or migraine headaches. A telephone discussion between the ED triage nurse and the charge nurse in the labor and delivery unit may be the best method of determining whose expertise is most needed for the evaluation and care of the maternal–fetal dyad.

When a woman of more than 20 weeks of gestation presents to the ED with cardiovascular, respiratory, or orthopedic complaints, the maternal and fetal vital signs should be assessed and documented. Appropriate ED screening questions, regardless of the reason she presents for triage, include the following:

- Is your baby's movement today the same as in previous days?
- Are you having any cramping, pelvic pressure, backache, or contractions?
- Is there any vaginal bleeding or leaking of fluid?

A decision tree is useful for triage of the maternal–fetal dyad. Although ED staff may have algorithms to follow for geriatric, pediatric, and nonpregnant adult patients, standard algorithms specific for the pregnant woman are uncommon. Some facilities develop their own written guidelines for appropriate care. To consistently meet the standards of care for a pregnant woman who presents to the facility for any reason, a triage decision tree should be developed by the ED and obstetrical nursing and medical staff. The triage decision tree should be used to determine whether the woman should remain in the ED or be transferred to surgery, critical care, or the labor and delivery suite (Figure 8-1).

The following chart is an example of a brief decision guide:

Woman of less than 20 weeks of gestation, regardless of concern	Emergency services department
Woman of more than 20 weeks of gestation with a pregnancy-related concern	Labor and delivery
Woman of more than 20 weeks of gestation with a nonpregnancy-related issue	ED with obstetrical consult

The phrase *obstetrical consultation* requires definition by each institution. It may mean fetal assessment or monitoring in the ED by an ED registered nurse who is competent in obstetrics, or it could mean that a labor and delivery nurse goes to the ED to evaluate the woman. Another option is to provide care in the ED and then transfer the woman to the labor and delivery unit for assessment by a perinatal nurse. Furthermore, *pregnancy-related* may be difficult to define. The fetus may be best served by having a labor and delivery caregiver evaluate the woman in the ED so that the woman and fetus are cared for simultaneously. This approach becomes more significant when trauma is involved.

A helpful tool for establishing institutional guidelines is *The Obstetrical Patient in the ED*, a joint position statement by the Emergency Nurses Association (ENA) and the Association of Women's Health, Obstetric, and Neonatal Nurses (AWHONN). Initiated in 1988, the statement has been revised (ENA, 2000) and can be located on the ENA website at www.ena.org.

Pregnant Trauma Victim Assessment and Care

Trauma is the leading cause of death in women of childbearing years, and it is the highest non-obstetrical cause of death during pregnancy. Trauma occurring in pregnancy is complicated. Trauma teams are often not accustomed to caring for pregnant women and their physiological adaptations specific to gestation, and obstetrical teams are unfamiliar with caring for trauma patients. Certain

Emergency Department of Triage Pregnant Patient

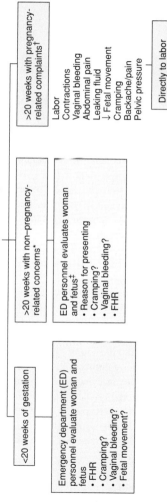

<20 weeks of gestation	>20 weeks with non–pregnancy-related concerns*	>20 weeks with pregnancy-related complaints†
Emergency department (ED) personnel evaluate woman and fetus • FHR • Cramping? • Vaginal bleeding? • Fetal movement?	ED personnel evaluates woman and fetus‡ • Reason for presenting • Cramping? • Vaginal bleeding? • FHR	Labor Contractions Vaginal bleeding Abdominal pain Leaking fluid ↓ Fetal movement Cramping Backache/pain Pelvic pressure
		Directly to labor and delivery (L&D)

*When a woman at >20 weeks of gestation arrives at the ED with an *emergency* medical condition (e.g., trauma), she is evaluated in the ED immediately, and the L&D nurse is called to come to the ED to assess and monitor the fetus and the pregnancy.

†The pregnant woman may present with headache, nausea and vomiting, epigastric pain, or visual changes, and these may be pregnancy related.

‡ED physician may ask L&D nurse to come to the ED for fetal monitoring when gestation is >24 weeks, *or* the pregnant woman may be sent to L&D triage for fetal assessment after being seen by the ED physician. L&D nurse reports triage assessment to obstetrician.

Figure 8-1
Emergency department triage of the pregnant woman.

injuries are unique to the pregnant trauma patient: uterine damage, placental abruption, and intrauterine fetal demise. The most common cause of fetal death is maternal death. Consideration of gestational age is an important factor. A decision must be made about the willingness to intervene operatively on behalf of the fetus. The lower limit of gestational age at which intervention may be carried out for the fetus may be as early as 24 weeks, when a fetus is considered potentially salvageable and viable. In addition, the impact of maternal trauma on the fetus may not be immediate. When there has been blunt abdominal trauma or when vaginal bleeding is present, the blood must be examined for fetal blood and the fetus monitored over many hours. It is inadequate in this situation to be reassured by a normal fetal heart rate tracing. Trauma concerns specific to pregnancy are in Table 8-1.

The *primary survey* of an injured pregnant woman addresses the same concerns (airway, breathing, circulation [the ABCs]) addressed for any other trauma victim, with the woman receiving priority over the fetus. Supplemental oxygen may be essential to prevent both maternal and fetal hypoxemia. Survival of the fetus depends on adequate uterine perfusion and the delivery of oxygen. Catecholamine release due to either anxiety or hemorrhage can cause uteroplacental vasoconstriction and can compromise fetal circulation. Avoiding the supine position optimizes maternal and fetal hemodynamics. Any diversion of blood flow from the uterus to maternal vital organs from hypotension will, depending on severity and duration, eventually lead to fetal tachycardia, a decrease in variability, late decelerations, and bradycardia *even before* there are changes in maternal vital signs. The placenta circulates 500 to 700 ml of blood per minute. Thus aggressive volume resuscitation is encouraged even when the woman is normotensive. The fetus acts as an internal pulse oximeter for the woman, as evidenced by fetal heart rate (FHR) patterns that reflect hypoxemia secondary to the maternal hypotension.

Emergency management of the pregnant trauma victim typically involves the following (Kass, Abbott, 2001):
■ Maternal resuscitation
■ Optimization of maternal oxygenation
■ Optimization of intravascular volume
■ Prevention or treatment of supine hypotension
■ Avoid hesitation about needed radiographic imaging
■ Intubate early if not oxygenating well

Table 8-1   Trauma concerns specific to pregnancy

Abruption

Result of "shearing" effect when uterus is deformed by external forces, causing separation from placenta	Can trigger diffuse intravascular coagulation because of high concentration of thromboplastin in placenta
	Electronic fetal monitoring is most sensitive means of detecting abruption
	Ultrasound most specific but lacks sensitivity
Vaginal bleeding poor predictor of abruption	May be a later sign; watch fundal height; increased uterine activity, increased pain

Uterine Rupture

Blunt trauma	Use ultrasound, x-ray; palpate fetal parts outside uterus; assess pain

Maternal–Fetal Hemorrhage

Four to five times more common in injured woman than in noninjured woman	Fetal anemia, death, or isoimmunization

Fetal Compromise

Nonspecific complication but most common	Late decelerations, tachycardia, loss of variability

Preterm Contractions

Common after blunt trauma	Abruption with potential for fetal hypoxia

Fetal Injuries

Skull fractures, intracranial hemorrhage	More common in third trimester

- Abdominal ultrasound evaluation for retroperitoneal hemorrhage
- Determination of fetal cardiac activity and gestational age
- Obstetrical consultation immediately after primary survey
- Electronic fetal monitoring when fetus is more than 24 weeks of gestation
- RhoGAM to all Rh-negative women who are known to be unsensitized

The *secondary survey* or assessment involves performing a physical examination, evaluating the pregnancy, and monitoring the fetus. The obstetrical history should cover the following:

- Last menstrual period (LMP) and estimated date of delivery (EDD) or of confinement (EDC)
- Problems and complications of the pregnancy
- Measurement of fundal height to approximate gestational age
- Presence of vaginal bleeding
- Evaluation for ruptured membranes
- Uterine activity
- Fetal heart rate and rhythm
- Fetal activity and movement
- Assessment of placenta for placental abruption with ultrasound
- A Kleihauer-Betke test from maternal blood to evaluate for maternal–fetal hemorrhage
- Apt test of vaginal blood to identify potential fetal origin

Fetal evaluation begins with an assessment of fetal movement and fetal heart rate. Doppler ultrasound may be used initially to locate and assess the fetal heart rate. Then, electronic fetal monitoring remains the most valuable adjunct tool for fetal evaluation in the gestation that is more than 24 weeks. Electronic monitoring of the fetus and uterine activity should be an integral part of the early and ongoing evaluation of the fetus, as it allows early recognition of the response to volume therapy or of sudden development of fetal jeopardy. In addition, uterine irritability or contractions observed on the tracing may provide clues to placental abruption, trauma, or uterine injury. Loss of variability and late decelerations or brady-cardias are the most sensitive findings in the detection of abruption (Abbott, 1999). Bedside ultrasonography can be useful to detect fetal cardiac activity and amniotic fluid volume, and, although the sensitivity for abruption is not good, it can help to evaluate subchorionic clots to see whether they are expanding or stable.

The Kleihauer-Betke test can estimate the volume of fetal blood in the maternal circulation but cannot predict other complications.

It should not replace fetal monitoring and ultrasound (Kass, Abbott, 2001). It may be helpful in determining the amount of immune globulin (RhoGAM) needed for the unsensitized Rh-negative woman experiencing trauma, but it should not be used to determine the *need* for RhoGAM.

The maternal circulation is protected at the expense of the fetal circulation during hypovolemia. Shunting within the fetus can compensate for hypoxia, protecting the woman's vital organs. Maternal tachycardia and hypotension occur late in shock and only after more than 30% of the maternal volume is lost. The vaso-constrictive effect of maternal hypoxia, acidosis, and sympathetic stimulation are often seen in hypovolemic shock and compromise the fetus's oxygen supply. The vascular bed does not autoregulate, and blood flow to the fetus varies with the maternal arterial pressure. Thus it is imperative to keep the woman normotensive to protect the fetus. The FHR pattern is a valuable tool for reflecting maternal cardiovascular and respiratory well-being.

There are two indications for emergent cesarean delivery: a live fetus that has demonstrated FHR patterns of compromise, and a moribund woman who does not respond to initial primary inter-ventions of trauma resuscitation (Luppi, 1999). As in cardiac arrest, delivery of the fetus may allow not only fetal resuscitation but also restoration of maternal venous return and perhaps a successful maternal resuscitation. A decision tree for the unstable pregnant trauma patient may be a useful resource (Figure 8-2).

The role of the intrapartum registered nurse who assists in caring for a pregnant woman with trauma includes the following:

- Assisted bag and mask ventilation (aggressive airway manage-ment is a necessity)
- Initiating intravenous access (having two sites is helpful)
- Administering medications
- Assessing fetal status
- Evaluating and ruling out fetal compromise
- Assessing uterine activity: contractions; low-amplitude, high-frequency (LAHF) contractions; or irritability associated with abruption
- Drawing blood and relating laboratory values to pregnancy norms
- Assisting with hemodynamic line placement
- Basic life support and manual uterine displacement
- Circulating at a postmortem cesarean delivery

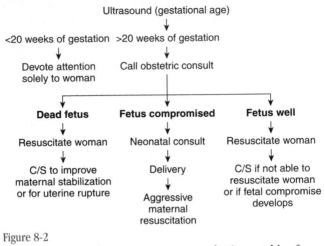

Figure 8-2
Decision tree for the pregnant woman who is unstable after trauma. C/S, Cesarean section.

- Reminding trauma team of the Ds in the ABCD of advanced resuscitation techniques: *d*isplacement (of the uterus), *d*efibrillate, *d*rugs, and *d*elivery (Johnson et al, 1999)

Once stabilized, a woman with trauma can often be transferred to the perinatal unit for continued care and monitoring. If she remains unstable, she may need to be transferred to surgery or to the intensive or critical care unit. The intrapartum or labor and delivery nurse should continue caring for the pregnant woman and her fetus regardless of where the woman has been transferred to from the ED. Again, where the assessment and care take place is not the concern. What is important is that the individual who is performing and interpreting information should be the most competent person to do so.

An issue that is raised with pregnancy and trauma is electronic fetal monitoring, which should be used for fetal and uterine assessment after trauma. There are no well-established standards for the duration of fetal monitoring after trauma (ACOG, 1998; Colburn, 1999). Many centers advocate 24 hours of continuous fetal monitoring. However, numerous studies have been done to determine risks that predict a poor outcome so that guidelines for electronic monitoring can be established (Biester et al, 1997; Shah, 1998). A pregnant woman who has sustained blunt abdominal trauma with any risk factors for preterm labor or abruption should be monitored for 24 hours. Those without these risk factors can safely be monitored for 6 hours and then discharged (Curet, 2000). If the fetus appears healthy on initial evaluation, frequent uterine contractions (more than eight per hour) in the first 4 hours is a sensitive, if nonspecific, predictor of later fetal complications and mandates a longer period of assessment. If the woman has no contractions or bleeding, and there is evidence of fetal movement on the fetal monitor tracing with reassuring parameters, 4 hours is probably a long enough evaluation period (Abbott, 1999). It is imperative to establish a baseline FHR, and any fetal tachycardia should be regarded with considerable suspicion. At discharge, the nurse should review with the woman the signs and symptoms of preterm labor along with the procedure for performing daily fetal kick counts, and give instructions for when to notify the health care provider.

Safety during pregnancy should be discussed prior to discharging a pregnant woman from the ED or the labor and delivery unit. Anatomic adaptations to pregnancy are associated with problems with coordination and balance, and falls are more common. Discussing safety features, proper body mechanics, and the avoidance of toxic chemicals may help the pregnant woman to avoid accidents. Instruction about appropriate seat belt use during pregnancy is an important aspect of discharge education. A combination lap belt and shoulder harness is the most effective auto restraint, and both should be used. The lap belt is worn low, underneath the uterus, and as snug as is comfortable. The shoulder harness is worn above the uterus and below the neck. The headrest can also prevent whiplash (Dobo, Johnson, 2000; Saunders, 2004).

Maternal–Fetal Transport Assessment and Care

First responders must understand the concepts presented in this chapter to provide appropriate care. It is vital that EMT, paramedic, and firefighter personnel promote maternal circulation and oxygenation and consider occult hemorrhage and shock in the pregnant trauma victim. All pregnant women should have supplemental oxygen and intravenous access established en route to the ED. If the pregnancy is of more than 24 weeks of gestation, alerting the hospital early during transport allows the staff to inform the obstetrical staff of the need for collaborative care immediately upon arrival. These first responders must understand the importance of transporting a pregnant woman of more than 20 weeks of gestation on her side or with a backboard tilt of 15 degrees to prevent supine hypotension (Kass, Abbott, 2001). Information regarding uterine status should be obtained and the woman asked about fetal activity. Vital signs should be assessed as often as they are for the nonpregnant woman, and uterine and fetal status should be evaluated whenever possible. Fundal height determination may be of great benefit in determining fetal age and the need for prompt obstetrical intervention on arrival to the emergency department. Simply noting the height of the uterus as above or below the maternal umbilicus can help determine if the pregnancy is more than or less than 20 weeks of gestation.

Non-Obstetrical Surgery: Maternal–Fetal Assessment and Care

It is estimated that 50,000 gravid women each year have surgery during their pregnancy (Kendrick, Powers, 1994; Inturrisi, 2000). The key points for caring for this dyad during surgery are collaboration and communication with all team members. During surgery, the goals for intact fetal survival include the following:

- Maintaining maternal blood pressure
- Maintaining maternal oxygenation
- Maintaining maternal circulating volume

No standard of care exists for assessing the fetus during non-obstetrical procedures, or for intervening on behalf of the fetus at early (less than 24 weeks) gestation. In fact, conflicting expert opinions exist regarding the necessity of intraoperative monitoring (Horrigan et al, 1999; Inturrisi, 2000). "The decision to use fetal monitoring should be individualized and, if used, may be based on gestational age, type of surgery, and facilities available" (ACOG, 2003). The advantages of monitoring for surgical procedures include enhanced communication among disciplines to focus on the safety of drugs for the fetus, patient positioning with regard to the effects on the fetus, altered maternal anatomy and physiology due to pregnancy, and the identification and need for an emergent cesarean delivery. Abdominal surgery commonly results in preterm contractions, which may evolve into preterm labor and birth.

Thus providers often consider administration of tocolytic agents before and after surgical procedures, especially abdominal procedures, that are likely to stimulate uterine activity (Inturrisi, 2000). These surgeries include placement of a renal stent, appendectomy, cholecystectomy, ovarian cyst and tumor removal, and trauma. Collaboration between the surgeon, anesthesiologist, and obstetrician ensures the safety of both patients and determines if intraoperative fetal assessment is necessary. Alerting the neonatal staff when the fetus is viable is also important for timely care for both patients.

Surgery When Gestation Is More Than 24 Weeks

When surgery is needed by a woman whose gestation is more than 24 weeks, the following points should be kept in mind:

- Preoperative cervical examination provides baseline information.
- Preoperative administration of a tocolytic medication such as Indocin can be helpful in preventing preterm contractions and uterine irritability.
- Preoperative medications are indicated to assist with gastric emptying and neutralizing gastric content, because of decreased gastric motility and relaxed gastric sphincters.
- Left uterine displacement after 20 weeks of gestation assists in avoiding hypertension and providing improved uteroplacental perfusion.
- Maintaining maternal oxygen saturation above 95% and maternal mean arterial pressure greater than 65 mm Hg helps keep the uterus perfused.
- Preoperative monitoring of the gravid uterus in a pregnancy of more than 24 weeks of gestation should be done with equipment appropriate for gestational age and by a nurse who is adept at both performing the procedure and interpreting the status of uterine activity and fetal heart rate patterns.
- Intraoperative monitoring (at >24 weeks) can be done with a Doppler or an ultrasound transducer (covered with as sterile sleeve) to reveal fetal compromise associated with maternal hypotension, interference with placental blood flow, manipulation of the maternal cerebrum, maternal hypothermia, or maternal hypoxia and acidosis.
- Postoperative monitoring of uterine activity and fetal assessment in the postanesthesia care unit (PACU) are continued as appropriate for gestational age, type of surgery performed, obstetrician's orders, and the presence or absence of uterine contractions.

- Surgery during pregnancy brings with it the risk of an urgent cesarean delivery. The neonatal staff should be notified and available for any neonatal emergencies that might arise. Depending on the surgery, an obstetrician may be present at the surgery or at least informed that the procedure is being performed (Inturrisi, 2000).

The parameters of fetal well-being (moderate variability and FHR accelerations) are not usually present during intraoperative monitoring because of the effects of anesthesia. Oxygen is rapidly consumed and cannot be stored by the fetus. Thus the fetus depends on a constant supply of oxygen. When a well-oxygenated fetus has an acute reduction in oxygenation, the decrease in blood flow falls below the fetal oxygen-carrying capacity to extract sufficient oxygen from the intervillous space. The fetal heart rate then shows evidence of this decrease in oxygen with late decelerations, an increase in baseline rate, and a decrease in variability.

The multidisciplinary approach to the pregnant surgical patient is optimal. Formulating a perioperative plan of care enhances the outcome for the maternal–fetal dyad. Communication between and involvement of all team members ensures the best possible outcome.

Federal Law and Triage

Triage incorporates a rapid assessment of the woman, identification of the concerns, determination of the acuity of the problem, and arrangement for the appropriate personnel and equipment to meet the woman's needs. Triage of all perinatal women is regulated by federal law via the Emergency Medical Treatment and Active Labor Act (EMTALA). This act requires that all hospitals provide a medical screening examination to determine if an emergency medical condition exists or if a woman is in labor. Prompt triage and a medical screening examination (MSE) must be performed in a timely manner, and if an emergency situation exists, treatment and stabilization are required prior to discharge or transfer (Mahlmeister, Van Mullem, 2000). The ENA and AWHONN support the development of hospital policies and procedures that specifically outline triage, care, and disposition of the perinatal woman. Their position statement referred to earlier in the chapter states that the care of a woman should take place in the area best prepared to handle her needs (ENA, 2000).

Summary

The initial emergent event and the physiological challenges of pregnant women require exceptional teamwork and communication combined with workable institutional protocols. Caregivers in the emergency department should understand fetal and maternal physiology to provide safe care to pregnant women. Collaboration between the ED and the labor and delivery staff is essential for developing guidelines and protocols.

References

Abbott J: Emergency management of the obstetric patient. In Burrow G, Duffy T, editors: *Medical complications during pregnancy*, ed 5, Philadelphia, 1999, Saunders.

American College of Obstetricians and Gynecologists (ACOG): Obstetric aspects of management: Trauma, *Educational Bulletin* no. 251, Washington, DC, 1998, The College.

American College of Obstetricians and Gynecologists: Non-obstetric surgery in pregnancy, *Committee Opinion* no. 284, Washington, DC, 2003, The College.

Biester E, Tomich P, Esposito T, Weber L: Trauma in pregnancy: Normal revised trauma score in relation to other markers of maternofetal status: A preliminary study, *Am J Obstet Gynecol* 176(6):1206 1212, 1997.

Colburn V: Trauma in pregnancy, *J Perinat Neonatal Nurs* 13(3):21-32, 1999.

Curet M, Schermer CR, Demarest GB, et al: Predictors of outcome in trauma during pregnancy: Identification of patients who can be monitored for less than 6 hours, *J Trauma* 49(1):18-25, 2000.

Dubo S, Johnson V: Evaluation and care of the pregnant patient with minor trauma, *Clin Fam Pract* 2(3):707-722, 2000.

Emergency Nurses Association (ENA), Association of Women's Health, Obstetric, and Neonatal Nurses (AWHONN): *Joint position statement: The obstetrical patient in the ED*, Des Plaines, Ill., 2000, Emergency Nurses Association.

Horrigan T, Villareal R, Weinstein L: Are obstetrical personnel required for intraoperative fetal monitoring during non-obstetrical surgery? *J Perinatol* 19(2):124-126, 1999.

Inturrisi M: Perioperative assessment of fetal heart rate and uterine activity, *J Obstet Gynecol Neonatal Nurs* 29(3):331-336, 2000.

Jevon P, Raby M, O'Donnell E: *Resuscitation in pregnancy: A practical approach*, Oxford, 2001, Butterworth Heinemann.

Johnson M, Luppi C, Over D: Cardiopulmonary resuscitation. In Gambling D, Douglas MJ (editors): *Obstetric anesthesia and common disorders*, Philadelphia, 1999, Saunders.

Kass L, Abbot J: Trauma in pregnancy. In Ferrera PC, Colucciello SA, Verdile V, Marx A editors: *Trauma management: An emergency medicine approach*, St Louis, 2001, Mosby.

Kendrick JM, Powers PH: Perioperative care of the pregnant surgical patient, *AORN J* 60(2):205-216, 1994.

Luppi C: Cardiopulmonary resuscitation in pregnancy. In Mandeville LK, Troino NH, editors: *High-risk and critical care: Intrapartum nursing*, ed 2, Philadelphia, 1999, Lippincott Williams & Wilkins.

Mahlmeister L, Van Mullem C: The process of triage in perinatal settings: Clinical and legal issues, *J Perinat Neonatal Nurs* 13(4):13-30, 2000.

Saunders R: Nursing care during pregnancy. In Lowdermilk DL, Perry SE, editors: *Maternity & women's health care*, ed 8, St Louis, 2004, Mosby.

Shah K, Simons RK, Holbrook T, et al: Trauma in pregnancy: Maternal and fetal outcomes, *J Trauma* 45(1):83-86, 1998.

Bibliography

Daddario J: Trauma in pregnancy. In Mandeville L, Troiano N, editors: *High-risk and critical care: Intrapartum nursing*, ed 2, Philadelphia, 1999, Lippincott, Williams & Wilkins.

Kendrick JM: Fetal and uterine response during maternal surgery, *MCN Am J Matern Child Nurs* 19(3):165-170, 1994.

Kendrick JM, Woodard CB, Cross SB: Surveyed use of fetal and uterine monitoring during maternal surgery, *AORN J* 62(3):386-392, 1995.

Antepartum Fetal Assessment

9

Evaluation of fetal well-being and maturity is essential in the management of the pregnancy at risk. Generally, routine fetal surveillance through antepartum monitoring and testing is initiated because of the appearance of a nonreassuring sign or a problem that places the woman at risk (ACOG, 1999). The gestational age at which to begin surveillance varies by the indication, but usually the fetus has reached a viable gestational age.

Statistics indicate that more than two thirds of fetal deaths occur during the antepartum period (ACOG, 1999). Antepartum fetal assessment is used in pregnancies at risk for morbidity and mortality, and many surveillance tools are available. A strict protocol applicable to all women is not possible; however, a testing approach based on general principles and guidelines can be effective (Smith-Levitin, 1997; Freeman et al, 2003). This chapter will present current antepartum biophysical and biochemical assessment options.

Antepartum Testing

The goal of antepartum testing is to provide a means of detecting the risk of perinatal morbidity and to prevent fetal death. Health care providers working in antenatal testing must understand whom to test and how often, and the appropriate tool to use. This requires knowledge of maternal and fetal physiology, perinatal risk factors, and the limitations and benefits of each test. Pregnancies with risk factors (Table 9-1) include those that are complicated by maternal or fetal conditions that put the fetus at risk for uteroplacental insufficiency, hypoxia, and death (Smith-Levitin, 1997).

Registered nurses, advanced practice nurses, and physicians with professional expertise should keep up with technical developments in electronic fetal monitoring (EFM) in addition to interpreting fetal heart rate patterns. Nurses who perform fetal

Table 9-1   Indications for antepartum testing

Maternal	■ Chronic hypertension ■ Diabetes ■ Collagen vascular disease (systemic lupus erythematosus) ■ Cyanotic heart disease ■ Hyperthyroidism (poorly controlled) ■ Hemoglobinopathies (thalassemia syndromes) ■ Renal disease ■ Pulmonary disease (asthma) ■ Antiphospholipid syndrome
Fetal	■ Suspected intrauterine growth restriction (IUGR) ■ Isoimmunization (moderate to severe) ■ Fetal infections (listeria monocytogenes, toxoplasmosis gondii) ■ Decreased fetal movement ■ Multiple gestation ■ Cardiac malformation ■ Discordant twins
Pregnancy Related	■ Gestational diabetes, poorly controlled ■ Prior unexplained fetal death (or recurrent risk) ■ Postterm gestation ■ Pregnancy induced hypertension ■ Oligohydramnios ■ Polyhydramnios ■ Preterm premature rupture of membranes ■ Third trimester bleeding (after resolution of episode)

assessment during the antepartum period should receive both clinical and didactic instruction about the physiological interpretation of EFM. Skill evaluation should cover core competencies in auscultation, EFM, and assessment of uterine activity (AWHONN, 1998b). The Association of Women's Health, Obstetric, and Neonatal Nurses has published competencies and guidelines for nurses performing both electronic fetal monitoring and limited ultrasound.

In deciding when to begin testing, the first consideration is gestational age. Identification of fetal compromise before the age of neonatal viability is of no clinical value. Most at-risk pregnancies begin testing at 32 weeks of gestation or at the time the risk or concern presents itself. Seldom does testing begin before 26 to 28 weeks of gestation (ACOG, 1999).

Biophysical Assessment

Fetal Movement

In the neurodevelopment sequence, fetal movement begins at around 9 weeks of gestation, but the woman may not feel movements until 16 to 20 weeks. Perception of fetal movement is influenced by many factors, such as maternal size and parity. The rationale for using this test for surveillance is simple: the fetus that is hypoxemic decreases or stops moving to reduce oxygen needs.

Fetal movement kick counts are an easy, inexpensive, and noninvasive way to involve the woman in monitoring her fetus. They are also the oldest method of assessment and applicable to the largest group of women. Fetal movement counts have appeared in the literature since Biblical times, but not until 1970 were they studied scientifically. Studies have shown that fetal movement counts are an effective screening measure, with reported reductions in fetal mortality from 8.7 deaths per 1000 live births to 2.1 deaths per 1000 live births (Smith-Levitin, 1997). Fetal kick counts are the primary method of fetal surveillance for all pregnancies and should be taught to *all* obstetrical patients. All health care providers in an institution should have a concise and consistent teaching tool regardless of where they interact with the woman. The obstetrical office, the childbirth education center, the perinatal testing center, and the labor and delivery unit should all use the same instructions and documentation tools to avoid confusion and to assist women with compliance.

There are many ways to perform this test. Generally, the woman is asked to pick a time each day when her baby is the most active, to count for 1 hour, and to record the number of movements felt. Generally, the fetus is most active between 7:00 and 11:00 P.M. Figure 9-1 gives instructions for fetal kick counts with a sample log.

FETAL KICK COUNT: INSTRUCTIONS AND LOG
Six steps: how to use your counting log

1. Count movements anytime between 7:00 PM and 11:00 PM.
2. After you eat, lie down on your left or right side.
3. Mark down the **date** and **start time** on your log.
4. Place your hands over your abdomen and pay close attention to your baby's movements.
5. Every time your baby moves **or** kicks mark one of the boxes.
6. When the baby has moved **or** kicked 10 times write down the **stop time** on your log.
7. If you have not felt five movements, count again for another hour. If there are still less than five movements or kicks, call your provider or go to the labor and delivery unit of the hospital.

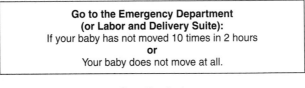

**Go to the Emergency Department
(or Labor and Delivery Suite):**
If your baby has not moved 10 times in 2 hours
or
Your baby does not move at all.

Counting Log

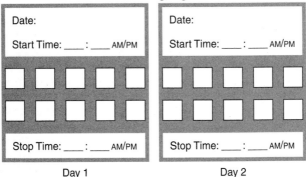

Date: _____

Start Time: ____ : ____ AM/PM

Stop Time: ____ : ____ AM/PM

Day 1

Date: _____

Start Time: ____ : ____ AM/PM

Stop Time: ____ : ____ AM/PM

Day 2

Figure 9-1
Fetal kick count instructions and log.
(Developed by the Women's Hospital Antepartum Testing Unit, LAC-USC Medical Center, Los Angeles, Calif. Courtesy Yolanda Rabello, RNC, MS Ed, CCRN.)

Nonstress Test
Description

The development of the nonstress test (NST) can be traced to an almost casual reference by Hammacher, who noted that the presence of accelerations with fetal movement represented an excellent indicator of fetal well-being (Schifrin, 1979). It is often the first test employed when a woman is referred for antenatal testing. The NST is based on the premise that a fetus that is not acidemic or neurologically depressed will demonstrate fetal heart rate (FHR) accelerations associated with fetal movement or uterine contractions, or in response to external stimuli. It is not necessary for the woman to perceive fetal movements in association with accelerations. If the reactive criteria are met, the test is reliable. A loss of reactivity, or absence of acceleration of the FHR, is most commonly associated with a sleep cycle but may result from central nervous system depression (e.g., from hypoxemia, drugs, or anomalies) (ACOG, 1999). There are no contraindications to this test.

Procedure for performing an NST

- Discuss the procedure with the woman.
- Position the woman in a semi-Fowler's position with a left lateral tilt.
- Perform Leopold's maneuvers and place both the ultrasound and toco transducers on the maternal abdomen (Figure 9-2).
- Fetal movement is recorded on the lower channel of the monitor strip. When the woman recognizes the movement, she depresses the event marker button of the fetal monitor, making a mark on the tracing. Some monitors print fetal activity blocks—the length of the block indicates the duration of fetal activity. The woman may also inform the nurse, who then makes a notation on the monitor strip. NOTE: It is not necessary for the woman to perceive fetal movements in association with accelerations in order to have an interpretable tracing.
- After 20 minutes, review the tracing. If criteria regarding a reactive test have been met, the test is complete even if fetal movement is not identified.
- If after 40 minutes the NST remains nonreactive, a vibroacoustic stimulus may be applied.

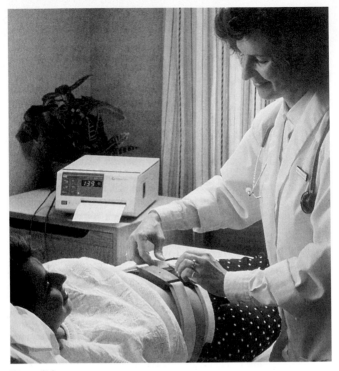

Figure 9-2
Application of external transducers to perform a nonstress test.
(Courtesy GE Medical Systems Information Technologies, Milwaukee, Wis.)

Interpretation

Reactive Test (Figure 9-3): The following guidelines can be followed to identify fetal reactivity. Minor variations in criteria are successfully used by various facilities.

- At least two accelerations with an amplitude of 15 beats per minute (bpm) above the baseline, with a duration of 15 or more seconds, within a 20-minute window
- Moderate FHR variability
- Absence of any nonreassuring periodic/episodic change

Nonreactive Test (Figure 9-4): Does not meet all of the criteria for a reactive test

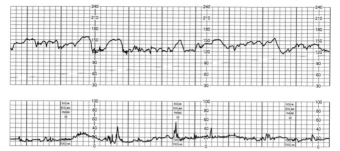

Figure 9-3
Reactive nonstress test (fetal heart rate acceleration; note fetal movement).

Clinical significance and management

A reactive NST suggests that the fetus will be born in good condition if labor occurs in a few days. The combination of an amniotic fluid index (AFI) with a nonstress test offers a more complete evaluation of fetal status.

The significance of a nonreactive NST should be further evaluated because the NST has a high false positive rate. With additional testing using the biophysical profile (BPP), most fetuses will show reassuring signs, and then a repeat NST can be scheduled when appropriate for the clinical situation. When the NST is used for primary surveillance, it should be performed twice weekly (ACOG, 1999).

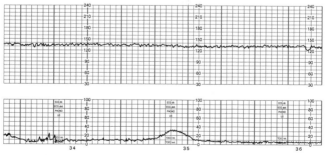

Figure 9-4
Nonreactive nonstress test (no fetal heart rate accelerations).

An inverse relationship exists between reactivity and gestational age, and by 28 weeks only about 50% of normoxic fetuses have a reactive nonstress test (Baker, 2000). However, *once a fetus has demonstrated the ability to achieve a reactive NST, regardless of gestational age, this ability should continue in the absence of compromise* (Menihan, 2000).

Vibroacoustic Stimulation

Description

Using vibroacoustic stimulation (VAS; also called the fetal acoustic stimulation test [FAST]) is a safe way to decrease false nonreactive nonstress tests and to shorten testing time without compromising detection of the acidemic fetus (Tan, Smyth, 2001). VAS is accomplished with an artificial larynx, which is available as an attachment to a fetal monitor or is obtained as a separate device. It generates sound levels of approximately 80 to 100 decibels. The combination of sound and vibration causes the fetal startle reflex and stimulation, which leads to accelerations of the FHR in the well-oxygenated fetus. Often with VAS, "less is more." A prolonged acceleration accompanying the stimulation can be confused with a baseline change and may appear to be tachycardia. The FHR should return to baseline before the woman is discharged. It is also important to note that the response to VAS may depend on gestational age and, prior to 30 weeks of gestation, the response to the stimulation may be absent (Tan, Smyth, 2001). In the presence of oligohydramnios, VAS has not been as successful in eliciting accelerations. For this reason, it is not always useful in the intrapartum period as an indirect method of assessing fetal acid–base balance. It is preferable that VAS not be done at the time of a cervical examination or during a uterine contraction.

Procedure

- Explain the procedure to the woman.
- Monitor the FHR and the uterine activity to obtain an interpretable tracing.
- Allow the woman to feel the stimulator on her hand so she understands it is not harmful to her fetus.
- Place the stimulator on the woman's abdomen over the fetal vertex and apply the stimulus for 1 second.
- Observe the monitor tracing for an acceleration of the FHR.
- A second stimulation may be applied if no acceleration occurs after 1 minute.

- Observe the tracing for an acceleration for 1 minute after the second stimulus.
- If no acceleration occurs after the second stimulus, apply a third stimulus for 2 seconds and wait for one additional minute for a response.

Interpretation

Reactive Test: Acceleration of the FHR, with an amplitude of 15 bpm above the baseline for a duration of 15 seconds

Nonreactive Test: Does not meet the criteria for a reactive test

Clinical significance

Stimulation of the fetus may be accomplished with vibroacoustic stimulation (VAS), and at times by gentle Leopold's maneuvers or noise. Regardless of how accelerations are elicited, once obtained they are a sign of fetal well-being. The tracing should be continued for up to 40 minutes before deciding the test is nonreactive. This accommodates the normal fetal sleep–wake cycles. If the fetus continues to be nonreactive, a biophysical profile is indicated.

Contraction Stress Test
Description

The basis for the CST is that a healthy fetus can tolerate a decreased oxygen supply during the physiological stress of a uterine contraction, whereas a compromised fetus will demonstrate late decelerations that are indicative of uteroplacental insufficiency. Variable decelerations may also occur in response to the contractions and suggest oligohydramnios (ACOG, 1999).

The CST can be performed by breast and nipple stimulation or by administering an exogenous source of oxytocin with an intravenous infusion. This is known as the oxytocin challenge test (OCT). Nipple stimulation is, of course, less invasive and less expensive. Careful evaluation of the fetal heart rate tracing is imperative with both techniques, as hyperstimulation of uterine activity may occur with either method.

Although the NST can be performed on any woman, the CST cannot. The potential for preterm labor precludes performing the test on women with certain risk conditions and gestational ages. The CST is contraindicated when any of the following situations exist:

- Premature rupture of membranes
- Placenta previa
- Third-trimester bleeding

- Previous classical cesarean scar
- Multiple gestation
- Incompetent cervix
- Risk for preterm delivery

Procedure for nipple-stimulated contraction stress test

Procedure	Rationale
1. Assist the woman to a semi-Fowler's position with a lateral tilt.	1. To maximize uteroplacental blood flow by avoiding supine hypotension
2. Place the tocotransducer where the least maternal tissue is in evidence—usually above the umbilicus.	2. To ensure that the fundus is as close as possible to the pressure-sensing device
3. Place the ultrasound transducer on the maternal abdomen where the clearest fetal signal can be obtained.	3. To ensure that the tracing is clear and interpretable
4. Monitor baseline FHR and uterine activity until 10 minutes of interpretable data are obtained (defer nipple stimulation if three spontaneous unstimulated contractions of more than 40 seconds' duration occur within a 10-minute period).	4. To provide a basis for comparison (it may not be necessary to proceed with test if spontaneous contractions occur)
5. Instruct woman to brush palmar surface of the fingers over the nipple of one breast through her clothes; continue four cycles of 2 minutes on and 2 to 5 minutes off; stop when contraction begins and restimulate when contraction ends (if a 2-minute period has elapsed).	5. To stimulate oxytocin secretion into the circulation from the pituitary gland
a. If unsuccessful after four cycles, restimulate the breasts for 10 minutes, stopping when contraction begins and resuming when contraction ends.	a. To maintain uterine contractions

Procedure	Rationale
b. If unsuccessful, begin bilateral continuous stimulation for 10 minutes, stopping when contraction begins and resuming when contraction ends.	
6. Discontinue nipple stimulation when three or more spontaneous contractions lasting longer than 40 seconds occur in a 10-minute period and are palpable to the examiner.	6. To eliminate unnecessary stress
7. Interpret results and continue monitoring until uterine activity has returned to the prestimulation state.	7. To ensure that the woman and fetus are restored to their prestress status

If nipple stimulation does not produce the desired uterine activity, an oxytocin-stimulated CST is indicated. Interpretation guidelines for CST are described after the oxytocin challenge test.

Oxytocin challenge test

The oxytocin challenge test is performed in the inpatient setting because labor may be stimulated in some sensitive women, particularly in those at term.

Procedure	Rationale
1. Assist the woman into a semi-Fowler's position with a lateral tilt.	1. To maximize uteroplacental blood flow by avoiding supine hypotension
2. Place the tocotransducer where the least maternal tissue is in evidence—usually above the umbilicus.	2. To ensure that the fundus is as close as possible to the pressure-sensing button
3. Place the ultrasound transducer where the clearest fetal heart sound can be heard—usually below the umbilicus.	3. To obtain a clear fetal signal

Procedure	Rationale
4. Monitor baseline FHR and uterine activity until 10 minutes of interpretable data are obtained before administration of oxytocin.	4. To provide a basis for comparison
5. Check the woman's blood pressure and pulse (following facility policy).	5. To identify hypotension resulting from maternal position
6. If less than three spontaneous unstimulated contractions occur within a 10-minute period and if late decelerations do not occur with spontaneous contractions, oxytocin can be initiated.	6. Oxytocin stimulation may not be necessary if adequate uterine activity is present. *The test is discontinued if late decelerations occur with spontaneous contractions.*
7. Piggyback oxytocin into the primary IV line (with lactated Ringer's or other nonaqueous solution) in the port nearest the IV insertion site.	7. May be necessary to stop oxytocin and rapidly infuse the primary IV in the event of uterine hyperstimulation or maternal hypotension
8. Administer oxytocin, beginning with 0.5 to 2.0 mU/min, with a constant infusion pump per facility protocol.	8. To ensure specific dosage of oxytocin
9. Increase the dosage of oxytocin infusion by 0.5 to 1.0 mU/min at 15-minute intervals until the contraction frequency is three in 10 minutes of 40 seconds' or more duration and contractions are palpable to the examiner.	9. To ensure a safe rate of oxytocin increments; generally the dosage of oxytocin does not exceed 5 mU/min, but on rare occasions doses of up to 10 mU/min may be necessary.
10. Discontinue the oxytocin when three contractions have occurred within a 10-minute period of interpretable data.	10. To provide enough stress to allow an interpretation

Procedure	Rationale
11. Discontinue the oxytocin any time there is evidence of hyperstimulation, prolonged bradycardia, or consistent late decelerations; treat non-reassuring FHR patterns in the same manner as during intrapartum monitoring; be prepared to administer terbutaline for tocolysis.	11. To prevent additional fetal stress; the principles for treating a nonreassuring FHR apply during both antepartum and intrapartum monitoring.
12. Continue to monitor until uterine activity and FHR return to baseline status.	12. To ensure that the woman and fetus are restored to their prestress status

Interpretation of the CST

Negative Test: Absence of late decelerations or significant variable decelerations with three contractions in a 10-minute window (Figure 9-5)

Positive Test: Late decelerations occurring with *more* than 50% of the contractions, regardless of contraction frequency (Figure 9-6)

Equivocal/Suspicious: Late decelerations occurring with *less* than 50% of contractions, or significant variable decelerations

Equivocal/Hyperstimulation: Late decelerations occurring with uterine contractions that are more frequent than every 2 minutes,

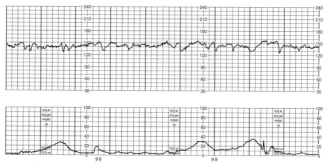

Figure 9-5
Negative contraction stress test (reassuring external fetal heart rate tracing).

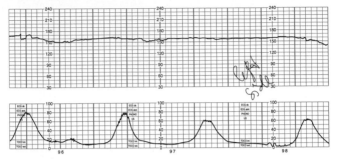

Figure 9-6
Positive contraction stress test (nonreassuring late decelerations with uterine contractions).

or a frequency of six or more UCs in 10 minutes, or contractions lasting longer than 90 seconds

Unsatisfactory Test: The frequency of three uterine contractions cannot be obtained in a 10-minute window, or the quality of the recording is not sufficient to be accurately interpreted

Clinical significance and management

The CST is highly reliable when it is negative and is reassuring that the fetus is likely to survive labor should it occur within a week. False negatives are rare unless hyperstimulation patterns are unrecognized or when the maternal position is supine, which results in hypotension and late decelerations. Fetal assessment utilizing other techniques such as the BPP may be indicated in some women. In other women, immediate termination of pregnancy may be warranted. Should a woman in labor with a previous positive CST have no late decelerations, it is likely to be the result of a correction of uteroplacental insufficiency in the interval between the test and labor.

Ultrasound

Ultrasound has many uses in obstetrics. There are three levels: limited, basic, and comprehensive (ACOG, 1993) (Table 9-2). A properly educated and credentialed nurse who has completed both didactic and clinical training may perform most of the components of the limited ultrasound. The *limited* ultrasound examination is used to determine amniotic fluid volume, to obtain

Table 9-2   Levels of ultrasound examination

Basic	Fetal number, presentation, fetal cardiac activity, placental location, amniotic fluid index, gestational age, fetal anatomy for gross malformations, maternal pelvic masses
Limited	Fetal number, presentation, fetal cardiac activity, placental location, biophysical profile, amniotic fluid index.* The following additional components are performed by the obstetric healthcare provider: ultrasound-guided amniocentesis, external cephalic version, localization of placenta in antepartum hemorrhage
Comprehensive	Examination of specific anatomic structures; may include an echocardiogram; performed by a sonologist or maternal–fetal specialist

*RNs who are credentialed to perform limited ultrasound may perform these components.

the biophysical profile, to identify fetal cardiac activity, to confirm fetal presentation, and to perform procedures such as an external version and amniocentesis. The *basic* ultrasound examination, the most common in pregnancy, is used to identify fetal number, presentation, cardiac activity, placental location, amniotic fluid volume, gestational age on the basis of standardized fetal biometrics (Figure 9-7), anatomic malformations, and the maternal adnexa. If any abnormalities are suspected on the basis of previous examinations, history, or physical examination, the woman is then referred to an examiner, usually a perinatologist, with expertise in *comprehensive* ultrasound.

Nurses who perform ultrasound examinations are accountable for the quality and accuracy of their assessment and for the information obtained from the examination (Stringer et al, 2003). It is of concern that bedside nurses without appropriate education and training are accepting the responsibility in the clinical setting for performing ultrasound (e.g., to determine fetal position, locate the fetal back for placement of the ultrasound for fetal monitoring) without having the appropriate competency (Menihan, 2000). Guidelines for the use of limited ultrasound by nurses have been developed by AWHONN (1998a) and provide a resource with

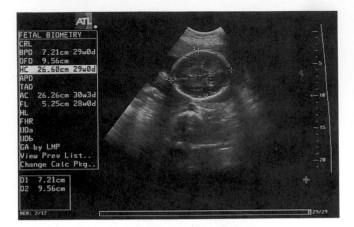

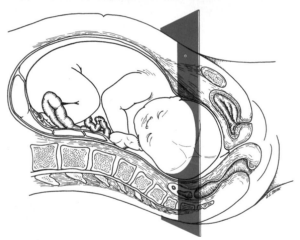

Figure 9-7
Schema of transverse section illustrates ultrasonographic view
of fetal head.

recommended educational and clinical activities to promote
competency (AWHONN, 2000).

Biophysical principles

Ultrasound is sound waves beyond the range of human hearing.
Sound is measured in hertz (Hz), which denotes cycles per second.

The frequency range of human hearing is from 20 to 20,000 Hz. The frequency range used in diagnostic ultrasound is 2 to 10 mega (million) hertz (MHz) and is determined by the transducer, which converts electrical energy into sound waves. The transducer contains crystals, or elements, that have piezoelectric properties. The word *piezoelectric* is derived from the German for "pressure electric." Crystalline quartz, lithium sulfate, lead zirconate, and barium titanate have piezoelectric properties—the ability to convert mechanical pressure into electrical energy, and vice versa. The crystal is struck electrically to produce a mechanical pulse. When ultrasound produced by the crystal traverses an object at a 90-degree angle (i.e., perpendicularly), the echoes returning to the crystal probe are recorded as dots of light on a cathode ray oscilloscope screen. The intensity and brightness of the dots correspond to the density and acoustic impedance, or resistance, met by a searching beam of sound at the various tissue interfaces. By moving the transducer in a specific scanning motion, the echoes from each tissue interface coalesce to trace the anatomic outline of that region.

Instrumentation technology has improved significantly since the inception of routine ultrasonography. The ultrasound transducer most commonly used in the obstetrical and gynecological setting is a curved, linear array, real-time transducer with a frequency of 3.5 to 7.0 MHz. This produces images faster than the eye can perceive, so the image appears to be in real time. The choice of the transducer frequency depends on the depth that must be penetrated. The faster the frequency, the shallower is the depth of penetration but the better is the resolution of the received echoes. In most term or near-term pregnancies, 3.5 MHz is necessary to visualize the entire uterine depth (Figures 9-8 to 9-10).

Safety

A safe level of ultrasound intensity has been defined, and most diagnostic ultrasound instruments produce energies far below that level. Ultrasound exposures at these intensities have not been found to cause any harmful biological effects on women, fetuses, or instrument operators in over three decades of research. However, because there is a potential for future identification of risks, it is recommended that ultrasound be used prudently and only when there is an indication (AIUM, 1998).

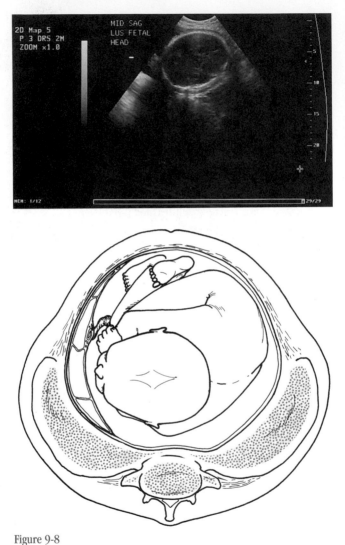

Figure 9-8
Ultrasonogram contrasted with corresponding schema of cephalic presentation in transverse section.

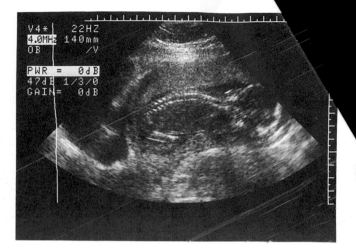

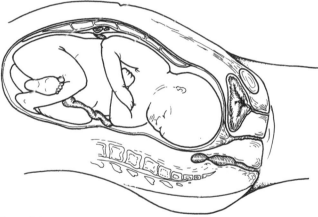

Figure 9-9
Ultrasonogram contrasted with corresponding schema of
cephalic presentation in longitudinal section.

Amniotic Fluid Index

During the second and third trimesters, amniotic fluid reflects fetal
urine production, and there is a 95% turnover every day. Placental
dysfunction may cause diminished fetal renal perfusion, which can

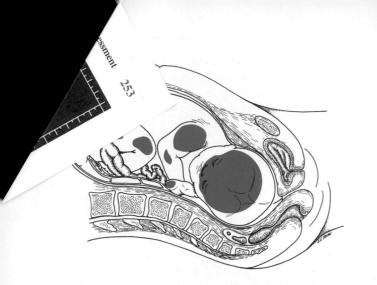

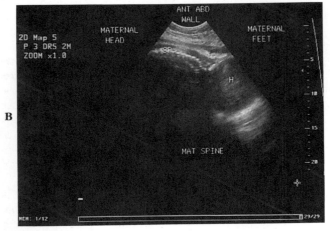

Figure 9-10
A, Schema of longitudinal section illustrates fetal head, body, and extremity in ultrasonogram. **B,** Longitudinal view of fetus with head toward maternal feet.

lead to oligohydramnios (Preboth, 2000). Oligohydramnios unrelated to fetal anomaly may precede the finding of intrauterine growth restriction (IUGR) (ACOG, 1999). If a low amniotic fluid index (AFI) is found before growth is affected, it is postulated that lifestyle changes such as increased maternal rest, or cessation of smoking, assist with increasing the AFI. More convincing data is needed to support a possible preventative effect on morbidity.

Oligohydramnios, pathological conditions, and impediments of the vessels in the umbilical cord increase the likelihood of variable or prolonged decelerations during antepartum testing. A fetus with *asymmetrical* IUGR has a normal head dimension but a small abdominal circumference. The fetus will protect vital organs (heart and brain), resulting in less perfusion to the nonvital areas of the body, including the kidneys. Small abdomens, thin limbs, and little fat are seen on these fetuses. This type of growth restriction is usually the result of placental nutritional insufficiency and is a *chronic* form of fetal stress (Peleg, 1998). In contrast, with an *acute* fetal stress (e.g., after abruptio placentae), the amniotic fluid volume will be unaffected because there has not been time to decrease fetal urine output.

In postterm pregnancies, the high frequency of FHR decelerations associated with decreased amniotic fluid volume suggests that the umbilical cord is vulnerable to compression and may be the mechanism of deterioration in fetuses remaining in the uterus. When conservative management is chosen, results seem best when the clinician carefully attends to fetal heart rate decelerations as well as to the amount of amniotic fluid volume. When any antepartum test shows fetal heart rate decelerations or decreased amniotic fluid volume, the postterm woman should be delivered.

In the presence of oligohydramnios, further evaluation is warranted regardless of the composite score of the BPP (Preboth, 2000). Sometimes a woman presents for antenatal testing and either oligohydramnios or polyhydramnios is found. Both of these findings need follow-up with a high-level ultrasound to rule out anomalies of the central nervous system, gastrointestinal system, or genitourinary system (ACOG, 1999).

Polyhydramnios can be associated with congenital anomalies or insulin-dependent diabetes, but most often the etiology is unknown. However, these women are at increased risk and should undergo antepartum testing. Some women with polyhydramnios will have problems with preterm contractions. Providers may choose to treat the fetus of less than 32 weeks of gestation with polyhydramnios with a regimen of indomethacin (Indocin). This drug decreases urine output in the fetus, thereby decreasing amniotic fluid volume. It is also a useful medication for the treatment of preterm labor. However, premature closure of the ductus arteriosus is a concerning and potential result of this medication; therefore the pregnancy should be followed with real-time ultrasound to continue monitoring the amount of amniotic fluid.

Women with insulin-dependent diabetes who have placental insufficiency may demonstrate an AFI within normal limits because their increased glucose levels result in increased fetal urine production and output. Thus a low amniotic fluid level in these fetuses may not be seen. In these cases, special attention must be paid to electronic fetal monitor tests, ultrasound imaging, fetal movement, and maternal insulin needs. These women normally have increasing insulin needs as the placenta comes into full maturity. At this point, insulin needs stabilize. In the third trimester, a careful assessment of the fetus is required if there is a trend toward decreasing maternal need for insulin, as this may correspond to decreasing placental function.

Prematurity generally does not affect fetal tone or amniotic fluid. In other words, a normal BPP score is expected even in the presence of prematurity (Baker, 2000).

Measurement of the amniotic fluid index

Procedure	Rationale
Assist the woman into the low semi-Fowler's position.	To avoid hypotension, and to have enough exposure of the abdomen for placement of ultrasound transducer on the appropriate area of the abdomen
Divide the uterus into four equal quadrants. At term, using the umbilicus, draw an imaginary line across the vertical axis, and using the linea nigra, draw an imaginary longitudinal line up and down the abdomen.	To divide the abdomen into four equal quadrants (Figure 9-11)
Holding the ultrasound trans-ducer in the longitudinal plane	To avoid measuring fluid from an adjacent quadrant by

Procedure	Rationale
and perpendicular to the floor, view each quadrant separately. Using calipers, measure the deepest pocket of fluid in each quadrant. Exclude umbilical cord and fetal parts from measurements (Figure 9-12).	appropriate placement of the transducer. In addition, keeping the transducer perpendicular avoids an oblique measurement of the pockets, which would result in a falsely increased apparent size of the pocket.
Add all values obtained.	To determine the amniotic fluid index

Amniotic fluid index values

>24 cm	Increased
10-24 cm	Normal
5.1-9.9 cm	Low-normal
≤ 5 cm	Decreased

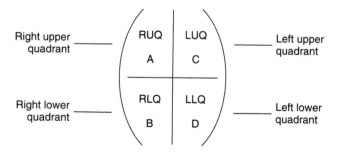

Four Quadrant Approach to AFI

Quadrants of the maternal abdomen

Figure 9-11

Four-quadrant approach to measurement of amniotic fluid index (AFI), which is calculated by adding the largest vertical pockets of amniotic fluid from each of the four quadrants of the gravid uterus.

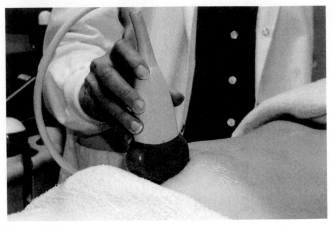

Figure 9-12
Proper position for holding ultrasound transducer in the longitudinal plane and perpendicular to the floor for measurement of amniotic fluid.
(Courtesy Meichelle Arntz, RNC, Santa Barbara, Calif.)

Interpretation and management

Increased AFI (>24 cm): Increased AFI is an indication for antepartum testing, including serial AFI measurements weekly. A complete ultrasound examination should be conducted to evaluate for associated fetal and placental abnormalities and for polyhydramnios.

Normal AFI (10 to 24 cm): Normal AFI is a reassuring finding during fetal testing.

Low-normal AFI (5.1 to 9.9 cm): Low-normal AFI should be evaluated with the gestational age in mind. Because amniotic fluid volume peaks at 34 to 35 weeks, an AFI of less than 10 cm should be reevaluated by additional measurements for the presence of associated conditions such as IUGR. A borderline value (5.1 to 7 cm) should be reevaluated every 3 to 4 days if all other findings are normal.

Decreased AFI (≤5 cm): Decreased AFI values in a woman at term or postterm indicates the need for delivery. When no amniotic fluid is found, a complete ultrasound examination should be conducted to rule out fetal anomalies. Rupture of the membranes may be a cause for decreased or absent amniotic fluid.

Biophysical Profile

The BPP involves evaluating the fetus with both electronic fetal monitoring and real-time ultrasound. The BPP measures five variables:

1. Fetal breathing movements
2. Gross body movements
3. Fetal tone
4. Fetal heart rate reactivity
5. Amniotic fluid volume

There are acute biophysical markers that are believed to be initiated and regulated by complex, integrated mechanisms of the CNS. Normal biophysical activity is indirect evidence that the portion of the CNS that controls specific activity is intact. The absence of this parameter is difficult to interpret, however, as it may reflect pathology or normal fetal periodicity. Amniotic fluid index is a marker of chronic fetal condition. Investigators have found an inverse relationship between NST and AFI findings—that is, the lower the AFI, the greater is the incidence of nonreactive NSTs and FHR decelerations.

A biophysical profile is often used to gather additional information when an NST is nonreactive, when a CST is positive, or for the preterm fetus that has not yet demonstrated the ability to accelerate the heart rate to an amplitude of 15 bpm for a duration of 15 seconds.

The biophysical profile, and all other aspects of limited ultrasonography, should be performed only by a provider who has demonstrated skill and competency after the completion of a didactic course with a clinical component. Liability is increased when a nurse conducts procedures outside of the scope of practice without the proper education, training, and documentation of competency.

Procedure

- Place the woman in a supine or semi-Fowler's position with a left lateral tilt. During the AFI, the woman will lie flat (Figure 9-13).
- Apply transducer gel or lotion to the woman's abdomen and note the time.
- Observe fetus with real-time ultrasound continually for a maximum time of 30 minutes. If all parameters of the test are met *prior* to 30 minutes, the test is then complete.
- Observe fetus for fetal breathing, fetal movement, fetal tone, and an AFI.

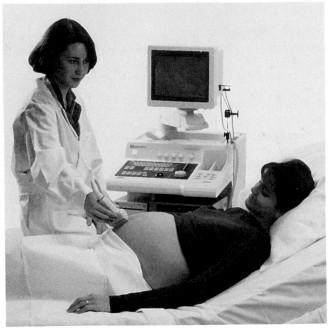

Figure 9-13
Nurse performing measurement of the amniotic fluid index.
(Courtesy GE Medical Systems Information Technologies, Milwaukee, Wisc.)

Interpretation

The following chart shows BPP scoring.

Biophysical Variable	Normal (Score = 2)	Abnormal (Score = 0)
Fetal breathing movements (FBM)	At least one episode of FBM of at least 30-sec duration in a 30-min observation	Absent FBM or <30 sec of sustained FBM in 30 min
Fetal movements (FM)	At least three trunk/limb movements in 30 min	Two or fewer episodes of trunk/limb movements in 30 min

Biophysical Variable	Normal (Score = 2)	Abnormal (Score = 0)
Fetal tone (FT)	At least one episode of active extension with return to flexion of fetal limb or trunk; opening and closing of hand considered normal tone	Absence of movement or slow extension/flexion
Amniotic fluid index (AFI)	≥1 pocket of fluid >1 cm in two perpendicular planes	Pockets absent or pocket <1 cm in two perpendicular planes
Nonstress test (NST)	Reactive: two or more episodes of FHR acceleration ≥15 bpm in ≥15 sec in 20 min	Nonreactive

Management

Decisions about clinical management require consideration of gestational age, fetal maturity, and maternal status. The following chart shows guidelines for patient care management based on the BPP score:

Score	Action
10	Score indicates fetus at minimal risk; repeat modified BPP in 3 to 4 days as indicated.
8	Repeat in 3 to 4 days; deliver if oligohydramnios is present; repeat twice weekly for diabetic women.
6	Consider delivery if fetus ≥36 weeks or if oligohydramnios is present; if fetus is immature, repeat BPP in 24 hr.
4	Deliver unless very immature; repeat within 24 hr if <32 weeks.
2	Deliver.

Modified Biophysical Profile

The modified BPP combines the nonstress test with the amniotic fluid index. This test is as predictive of fetal status as other types of biophysical fetal surveillance and is much less invasive, expensive, and time consuming than the contraction stress test (ACOG, 1999). The modified BPP is reassuring if the NST is reactive and the AFI is greater than 5 cm. Both criteria must be met.

Umbilical Artery Doppler Velocimetry

Umbilical artery Doppler velocimetry is a noninvasive technique used to assess the hemodynamics of vascular impedance. Developments in technology have allowed assessment of flow patterns and velocities in a number of fetal arteries, the umbilical artery being the most widely studied. Doppler flow velocity has been adapted as a fetal surveillance technique. It has been observed that flow velocity waveforms in the umbilical artery of fetuses with normal growth differ from those of fetuses with IUGR. The umbilical flow velocity of a normally grown fetus has a high-velocity diastolic flow. In cases of IUGR, the umbilical artery diastolic flow is diminished; in extreme cases, the flow may be absent or reversed, which carries a high mortality rate (ACOG 1999; Preboth, 2000). Doppler waveforms reflect the current status of placental blood flow and give an up-to-the-minute appraisal. Disease causes destruction of the small muscular arteries in placental tertiary-stem villi. The severity of the problem will be reflected in the decreasing end-diastolic flow. Reverse end-diastolic flow demonstrates an advanced stage of placental compromise and is associated with the obliteration of 70% of the placenta's arteries. Umbilical artery Doppler may be obtained from any segment of the cord, but those taken closer to the placenta reflect more diastolic flow than those at the fetal end. In practice, these differences are not clinically significant (Abuhamad, 2003).

Clinical Management Based on Results of Biophysical Testing

Timely communication with the primary health care provider is essential to ensure that nonreassuring test results are responded to in an appropriate way and lead to proper management of the woman and her fetus (AWHONN, 2000). There should be a mechanism in place to allow the primary health care provider an opportunity to view the EFM tracing and all test results. If results are abnormal, a phone call to the primary health care provider and an immediate management plan are necessary. The results and EFM strips may be faxed to, or viewed on off-site monitor screens at, the primary caregiver's office, to ensure that all results are viewed by the physician in a timely manner.

Although a single protocol cannot be applied to every clinical scenario, some general principles apply (Figure 9-14). First, a screening test with abnormal findings should be followed promptly by a more sensitive and specific test to avoid acting on a false-positive result. For example, a woman with decreased fetal movement should undergo a nonstress test; if that test is nonreassuring, a biophysical profile or CST should follow. Second, a test with equivocal or suspicious results should be acted on (e.g., with long-term monitoring or induction of labor) or repeated, or another test, such as the BPP, should be initiated.

Once a decision is made to proceed to delivery, the route and exact timing of delivery should be looked at carefully. Induction of labor is not necessarily contraindicated when the antepartum tests suggest uteroplacental insufficiency. Delivery can often be safely delayed while the woman's medical condition is stabilized (e.g., by controlling hypertension or correcting metabolic abnormalities), or while corticosteroids are administered to accelerate fetal lung maturity, as long as maternal and fetal conditions are closely monitored (Smith-Levitin, 1997).

Biochemical Assessment

Amniocentesis

An amniocentesis is the penetration of the amniotic cavity through the abdominal and uterine walls for the purpose of withdrawing fluid for examination. This procedure was first described by Bevis (1952), who noted the varying amounts of bile pigments in amniotic fluid while assessing Rh-isoimmunized pregnancies. Amniocentesis has become a standard tool in the assessment of fetal well-being and maturity as well as in the diagnosis of genetic complications and concerns.

The procedure is performed under ultrasound guidance by insertion of a 20- to 22-gauge spiral-type needle transabdominally to withdraw between 5 and 20 ml of amniotic fluid (Figure 9-15). When genetic problems are suspected, amniocentesis is performed as soon as possible, usually between 16 and 22 weeks, for karyotyping and biochemical studies. Amniocentesis later in pregnancy is most often performed to assess fetal maturity. In cases of isoimmunization, the procedure may be performed repeatedly to

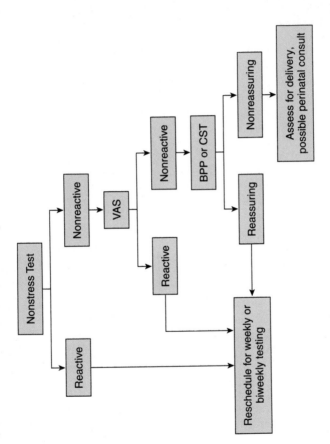

Figure 9-14
Algorithm for antepartum testing. *BPP*, Biophysical profile; *CST*, contraction stress test; *VAS*, vibroacoustic stimulation.

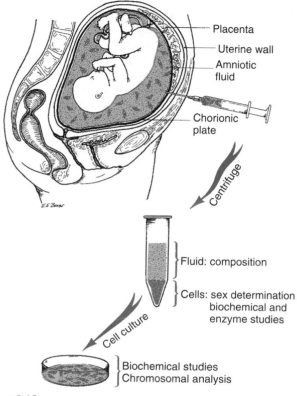

Figure 9-15

Amniocentesis. Amniotic fluid is aspirated with a sterile syringe. The sample is centrifuged to separate cells and fluid.

monitor the fetal condition. Amniocentesis is most often performed in the third trimester to assess fetal lung maturity for the most opportune time for delivery (ACOG, 1999).

There are minimal risks with amniocentesis. They include spontaneous abortion (when used in the second trimester), trauma to the fetus or placenta, bleeding, infection, preterm labor, and Rh sensitization from fetal bleeding into the maternal circulation. However, the risk of the procedure to the woman or the fetus is generally accepted to be about 0.5%.

Patient care

Assessment of fetal status should be performed both before and after the procedure, typically by a nonstress test. In some women, tocolysis may be needed prior to the procedure.

When the amniocentesis is completed, the woman should be observed for any untoward symptoms. If she feels faint, she should be assisted in turning to one side or the other to counteract any effects of supine hypotension. The fetus should be assessed after the procedure. The woman should be instructed to report any of the following to the physician should they occur after the procedure: vaginal drainage, uterine contractions, fever or chills, abdominal pain, and vaginal bleeding.

Fetal lung maturity

Some stressful conditions during pregnancy have been known to accelerate fetal lung maturity. They include preeclampsia, prolonged rupture of membranes, narcotic addiction, and intrauterine growth restriction. The acceleration may be the fetus's reflex response to a hostile intrauterine environment. In contrast, conditions in which fetal lung maturity tends to be delayed include diabetes mellitus and fetal hemolytic disease.

Acceleration of fetal lung maturity can be achieved when the glucocorticoid betamethasone is administered to the woman in whom preterm delivery is anticipated. The fetal lung maturation is reflected by a rise in the L/S ratio (described in next paragraphs), usually within 48 hours after initiating therapy. The greatest benefit is achieved if delivery occurs between 24 hours and 7 days after the initiation of treatment.

The assessment of fetal lung maturity is very important in managing delivery timing as it assists providers in preventing neonatal respiratory distress syndrome (RDS). The immature lungs may be unable to produce pulmonary surfactant, the lipoprotein that reduces surface tension in the water layer of the alveoli and that provides a coating that promotes inflation of the lungs. The five assessment tests currently in use for fetal lung maturity evaluation are accomplished by using amniocentesis to obtain a sample of amniotic fluid (ACOG, 1996, 1999).

Lecithin-to-sphingomyelin (L/S) ratio

Pulmonary surfactant contains primarily phospholipids. Surfactant acts as a surface detergent at the air–liquid interface of the alveoli, preventing their collapse at the end of expiration. The L/S ratio, considered the gold standard for determining lung maturity, compares the concentrations of the two phospholipids, lecithin and sphingomyelin, that are the major components of the surfactant complex. Normally during gestation, the sphingomyelin concentration is greater than that of lecithin, until about 26 weeks of gestation. From 26 to 33 weeks, the concentrations of lecithin and sphingomyelin are fairly equal (i.e., their ratio is 1:1). From 34 to 36 weeks, there is an increase in lecithin and the ratio rapidly rises. It is generally accepted that a ratio of 2.0 or greater indicates pulmonary maturity and that RDS will rarely occur. The following interpretation is generally accepted:

L/S Ratio	Fetal Lung	Risk for RDS
>2.0	Mature	Minimal
1.5-2.0	Transitional	Moderate
<1.5	Immature	High

This test does have disadvantages. It requires skill to perform, is slow, and is subject to contamination from blood or meconium, which results in false results.

Foam stability test

This test, also called the shake test, was developed by Clements and colleagues (1972) to decrease laboratory time needed to perform the L/S ratio. It is based on the ability of surfactant to generate a stable foam when ethanol is added to the amniotic fluid specimen. Ethanol, isotonic saline, and amniotic fluid at varying dilutions are shaken together for 15 seconds. At the proper dilution, a ring of bubbles at the air–liquid interface after 15 minutes indicates probable fetal lung maturity (Figure 9-16).

Phosphatidylglycerol

The assessment for the presence of phosphatidylglycerol (PG) is fast and relatively resistant to contamination by blood and

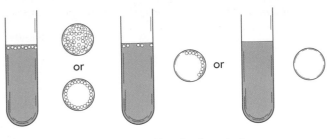

Positive foam test   Negative foam test

Figure 9-16
Clement's foam test (shake test). For the test to be positive,
bubbles must be seen around the entire circumference of tube.

meconium. The absence of PG indicates a high risk for RDS.
The interpretation of fetal lung maturity should not be based solely
on the presence or absence of PG, and this test is best used in
combination with the L/S ratio.

Fluorescence polarization (FLM-II assay)

The fetal lung maturity (FLM-II) assay uses fluorescence polarization to determine lipid membrane fluidity in amniotic fluid.
A fluorescence analogue is added to amniotic fluid and then
polarization is measured with a polarimeter. Surfactant has a low
polarization and albumin a high polarization. Interpretation of the
results for fetal lung maturity is shown in the following chart:

Mature	>55 mg/g
Transitional	40-54 mg/g
Immature	<39 mg/g

Lamellar body count

Lamellar body counting measures the number of surfactant-
containing particles in amniotic fluid directly by using the platelet
channel of a standard hematology cell counter. This is a quick
screening test (taking less than 10 minutes) for fetal lung maturity.
The rapidity is helpful in situations involving preterm labor,

premature rupture of membranes, worsening preeclampsia, or elective delivery at term. Lamellar bodies first appear between 20 and 24 weeks of gestation. Fetal breathing movements carry lamellar bodies into the amniotic fluid, where they can be counted. The phospholipid content and the laminated structure of the particles change with maturation of the fetal lung. By assessing the size and number of bodies in the amniotic fluid, fetal lung maturity can be predicted (Neerhof et al, 2001). Maturity is related to a reference interval as shown in the following chart.

Mature	$\geq$50,000/μL
Transitional	>15,000 to <50,000/μL
Immature	$\leq$15,000/μL

Treatment regimen

The treatment for fetal lung immaturity is two doses of betamethasone (12 mg given intramuscularly to the woman 24 hours apart) *or* four doses of dexamethasone (6 mg given IM 12 hours apart).

Pulmonary edema may occur in women who are being treated with a combination of corticosteroid therapy and beta-mimetic drugs. If there is premature rupture of membranes in a preterm gestation, the woman must be monitored closely for signs of infection (Anyaegbunam, Adetona, 1997).

Percutaneous Umbilical Blood Sampling

Percutaneous umbilical blood sampling (PUBS) provides direct access to the fetal circulation and is the most widely used method for fetal blood sampling and transfusion. It is also called *cordocentesis.* The addition of percutaneous umbilical cord blood sampling as an additional technique of fetal assessment has improved obstetric care in the isoimmunized patient because it provides a direct and precise measurement of fetal hematocrit and bilirubin. This is in contrast to amniocentesis, which provides an indirect measurement of fetal values. The knowledge of specific values permits the physician to determine the necessity and timing of fetal transfusions for isoimmunization. At times, results of percutaneous umbilical blood sampling may indicate an absence of the blood

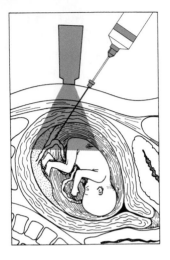

Figure 9-17
Technique for percutaneous umbilical blood sampling guided by ultrasound.
(From Lowdermilk D, Perry S, Bobak I: *Maternity & women's health care,* ed 7, St. Louis, 2000, Mosby.)

group antigen in question, and the fetus would not require any intervention nor further evaluation.

The procedure is achieved through the transabdominal insertion of a needle into the fetal umbilical vein under ultrasound guidance (Figure 9-17). The ideal puncture point in the umbilical vein is close to the insertion of the cord into the placenta. Between 1 and 4 ml of blood is removed and tested by the Kleihauer-Betke procedure to ensure that the specimen is fetal, not maternal, blood. The blood sample can be used for karyotyping, direct Coombs' test, complete blood count, fetal blood type, acid-base status, detection of infection, and detection of fetal anemia and the need for fetal blood exchange transfusion. Complications, which are unusual, include leakage from the puncture site, cord laceration, chorioamnionitis, thromboembolism, preterm labor, premature rupture of membranes, and fetal bradycardia. The procedure-related pregnancy loss rate has been reported to be less than 2% (ACOG, 2001).

Summary

Biophysical and biochemical means of antepartum surveillance play an important part in modern perinatal care and practice. It is essential that appropriate tests be chosen and properly conducted and the results appropriately acted on. Nurses play a vital role in this process and are often the caregivers conducting the testing. As with all aspects of perinatal care, communication and a collaborative approach to the assessment of the woman and fetus are the key to achieving the goal of improving perinatal outcomes and decreasing morbidity and mortality.

References

Abuhamad A: Does Doppler ultrasound improve outcomes in growth-restricted fetuses? *Contemp Ob/Gyn* 48(5):56-64, 2003.

American College of Obstetricians and Gynecologists (ACOG): Ultrasonography in pregnancy, *Technical Bulletin* no. 187, Washington, DC, 1993, The College.

American College of Obstetricians and Gynecologists: Assessment of fetal lung maturity, *Educational Bulletin* no. 230, Washington, DC, 1996, The College.

American College of Obstetricians and Gynecologists: Antepartum fetal surveillance, *Technical Bulletin* no. 188, Washington, DC, 1999, The College.

American College of Obstetricians and Gynecologists: Prenatal diagnosis of fetal chromosome abnormalities, *Practice Bulletin* no. 27, Washington, DC, 2001, The College.

American Institute of Ultrasound in Medicine (AIUM): *Bioeffects and safety of diagnostic ultrasound,* ed 2, Laurel, Md., 1998, The Institute.

Anyaegbunam WI, Adetona A: Use of antenatal corticosteroids for fetal maturation in preterm infants, *Am Fam Physician* 56(4):1093-1096, 1997.

Association of Women's Health, Obstetric, and Neonatal Nurses (AWHONN): *Clinical competencies and education guide: Limited ultrasound examinations in obstetric, gynecologic/infertility settings,* Washington, DC, 1998a, The Association.

Association of Women's Health, Obstetric, and Neonatal Nurses: *Nursing practice competencies and educational guidelines for examinations in obstetric and gynecology settings,* Washington, DC, 1998b, The Association.

Association of Women's Health, Obstetric, and Neonatal Nurses: *Fetal assessment: Position statement,* Washington, DC, 2000, The Association.

Baker B: Standard antepartum testing of preterm fetuses, *OB/GYN News* International Medical News Group, March 1, 2000.

Bevis DCA: The antenatal prediction of haemolytic disease of the newborn, *Lancet* 1:395-398, 1952.

Clements JA, Platzker AC, Tierney DF et al: Assessment of the risk of respiratory distress syndrome by a rapid test for surfactant in amniotic fluid, *New Engl J Med* 286(20):1077-1081, 1972.

Freeman RK, Garite TJ, Nageotte MP: *Fetal heart rate monitoring,* Baltimore, 2003, Williams & Wilkins.

Lowdermilk D, Perry S: *Maternity & women's health care,* ed 8, St Louis, 2004, Mosby.

Menihan C: Limited obstetric ultrasound in nursing practice, *J Obstet Gynecol Neonatal Nurs* 29(3):325-327, 2000.

Neerhof MG, Dohnal JC, Ashwood ER, et al: Lamellar body counts: A consensus on protocol, *Obstet Gynecol* 97(2):318-320, 2001.

Peleg D: Intrauterine growth restriction: Identification and management, *Am Fam Physician* 77(7):786-787, 1998.

Preboth M: Practice guidelines: ACOG guidelines on antepartum surveillance, *Am Fam Physician* 62(5):1189-1190, 2000.

Schifrin BS: The rationale for antepartum fetal heart rate monitoring, *J Reprod Med* 23(5):213-221, 1979.

Smith-Levitin M: Practical guidelines for antepartum surveillance, *Am Fam Physician* 56(8):1981-1988, 1997.

Stringer M, Miesnik SR, Brown LP, et al: Limited obstetric ultrasound examinations: Competency and cost, *J Obstet Gynecol Neonatal Nurs* 32(3):307-312, 2003.

Tan K, Smyth R: VAS for facilitation of tests of fetal well-being, *Cochrane Database Syst Rev* 1:CD002963, 2001.

Care of the Monitored Patient

10

The use of electronic fetal monitoring for antepartum and intrapartum women is a standard of practice for both low- and high-risk pregnancies. It is the standard of care to use electronic fetal monitoring in pregnancies with risk factors that indicate the need for nonstress testing (NST) and contraction stress testing (CST) during the antepartum period. It is expected that nurses obtain clear tracings and interpret baseline characteristics and periodic and episodic changes. It is the standard of care for nurses to identify various patterns; document assessments, interpretations, and interventions; and notify the appropriate providers (e.g., obstetricians, neonatologists, midwives) in a timely manner. Failure to do otherwise is practicing below the standard of care and may increase the risk of liability.

One must keep in mind that the electronic fetal monitor, regardless of its level of sophistication, is only one of the tools used for fetal surveillance. A fetal heart rate (FHR) tracing should never be the only assessment of fetal well-being. Other assessment data that must be interpreted concurrently with the tracing include subjective data obtained from the woman and/or her family during the admission interview, objective findings acquired from physical examination of the woman, laboratory data, results of any ultrasound examinations, and other pertinent data obtained from the woman's prenatal record.

The care given to the continuously monitored woman in labor is the same as that given to any woman during labor, with additional consideration to those factors that relate directly to the monitor. The most important item by far is a thorough explanation to the woman and her partner and support people about the monitor—how it is used, how it is applied, and what is being evaluated. Many women are anxious about the status of the baby, concluding that something must be wrong that necessitates the monitor use. Some women fear the machine itself and are distracted by its mechanical noises and beeps. Others are afraid to move in bed for fear of dislodging the internal and external monitoring devices and are concerned that the scalp electrode and intrauterine pressure catheter (IUPC) may harm the baby.

The health care provider must focus on the way in which people of different cultures and ethnicities perceive life events, the health care system, and the birthing process. To be effective, patient care must be provided in a culturally sensitive manner.

The digital display of the FHR is frequently a source of anxiety. Because the electronic fetal monitor cannot print out every heartbeat, a sampling of the FHR is displayed, and often very low or very high numbers are observed. In addition, the signal quality indicator may fluctuate in color, from green (for the best tracing) to yellow and to red at times, as a result of fetal movement. Time should be allowed for the signal to stabilize before repositioning the ultrasound transducer. Women expressing concern should be told that variations in the displayed FHR and signal quality indicator are to be expected.

Often the monitor is reassuring to the woman. The audible beeps of the fetal heart sounds can be reassuring that all is well with the fetus. The sound serves as encouragement, especially during active labor, when some women are overwhelmed by discomfort and lose sight of the imminent birth of their baby. For women who feel discouraged about labor, it is often reassuring to see evidence of uterine contractions. Visualizing contractions can also help the support person guide the laboring woman through the contraction by using breathing, focus, and relaxation techniques.

The woman and her support person should be informed about the fetal monitor and the monitor strip tracing of the FHR and uterine activity (UA). They can distinguish between the FHR and the uterine activity panel without much difficulty. They observe changes in the monitoring pattern, such as those caused by fetal movement, and can be given appropriate explanations when variations in the FHR occur. After all, should an emergency arise, there are no real secrets about the urgency of the situation.

Whether a woman is continuously or intermittently monitored during labor, the care and issues involving documentation are the same; the monitor should not receive more attention than the woman (Figure 10-1). During the antepartum and intrapartum periods, the obstetrical nurse is responsible for a minimum of two patients, maternal and fetal. This necessitates the use of both maternal and fetal surveillance, which includes risk assessments determined through history taking, physical examination, and biochemical and biophysical testing. Laboring women are monitored for progress of labor, maternal well-being, pain management, psychosocial evaluation, and cultural needs. Intrapartum surveillance allows evaluation of fetal tolerance of labor and determines fetal well-being. Guidelines for care are described in the following quick-reference outline.

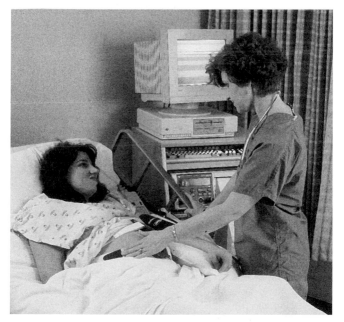

Figure 10-1
The nurse manages the care of an electronically monitored woman, ensuring that the monitor does not receive more attention than the woman.
(Courtesy GE Medical Systems Information Technologies, Milwaukee, Wis.)

Admission Assessment

- Review prenatal records, including history, laboratory, and ultrasound data, and the physical examination.
- Obtain vital signs, including temperature, respiration, pulse, and blood pressure.
- Review or perform vaginal examination, including cervical effacement, dilatation and station, and fetal presentation and position.
- Ask the woman about status of membranes. If rupture of membranes has occurred before admission, document date and time of rupture, and the amount, odor (if any), and color of the fluid.
- Inquire about the woman's preferences for pain management, her labor preferences, and her birth plan.
- Assess uterine activity, including contraction onset, frequency, duration, and intensity.
- Determine baseline fetal heart rate, variability, presence or absence of periodic or episodic changes.
- Provide information to the woman and her family about the electronic fetal monitor. This may include the reason for monitoring, where the transducers will be located on the abdomen, and what information can be obtained from them.
- Explain central monitoring and/or bedside electronic documentation.
- Other assessments and observations may be included in the admission assessment as the woman's condition warrants.

Care During First Stage of Labor

The first stage of labor consists of three phases: early labor, active labor, and transitional labor:

Early labor: Dilation of 0 to 4 cm with mild to moderate irregular contractions

Active labor: Dilation of 4 to 8 cm with moderate to strong regular contractions every 2 to 5 minutes

Transitional labor: Dilation of 8 cm to complete dilation (10 cm) with strong contractions

Assessment
Subjective data

Behavior
    Surge of energy and activity
    Talking frequently
    Anxious
    Fear of isolation

Objective data

Rupture of membranes
Uterine contractions: intensity, frequency, duration
Transitional labor
    Nausea and vomiting
    Hypersensitive abdomen
    Irritability
    Loss of coping mechanisms
    Hiccups and/or belching
    Trembling and/or shaking of legs
    Chills
    Perspiration
    Rectal pressure
    Urge to push

Potential complications

Nonreassuring maternal findings
    Fever
    Hypotension or hypertension
    Dehydration
    Circulatory overload
    Hemorrhage
    Severe pain unrelated to contractions
    Supine hypotension syndrome
    Distended bladder
Nonreassuring auscultated *or* electronically monitored fetal heart
    rate
    Fetal tachycardia: >160 beats/min
    Fetal bradycardia: <110 beats/min

Nonreassuring FHR in electronically monitored labor
    Severe variable decelerations: <70 beats/min for more than 60 seconds
        Rising baseline heart rate, decreasing variability, slow return to baseline
    Uncorrectable, repetitive late decelerations
        Decreasing variability or rising FHR baseline
    Minimal or absent variability
    Prolonged deceleration
    Severe bradycardia (<80 bpm)
    Unstable FHR; sinusoidal pattern
Inadequate uterine relaxation
    Contractions >90 sec
    Relaxation between contractions <30 sec
    Tachysystole (≥6 uterine contractions [UC] in 10 min)
    Hyperstimulation (≥6 UC in 10 min, with evidence of fetal intolerance)
Arrest of labor
    Protracted disorder (dilation <1.5 cm/hr)
    Arrest disorder (no change in dilation or descent in 2 hr)
    Prolonged latent phase
Meconium-stained amniotic fluid
Foul-smelling amniotic fluid
Fetal hyperactivity or hypoactivity
Intraamniotic infection secondary to prolonged rupture of membranes
Bleeding of unknown origin
Abruptio placentae
Uterine rupture

Multidisciplinary Management
Therapeutic management

- Laboratory tests as indicated
- Intravenous fluids as indicated
- Analgesia as indicated, per patient preference
- Preparation for selected/indicated anesthesia by anesthesiologist/nurse anesthetist
- Supportive care to the woman and family
- Education about labor, procedures, and interventions

Nursing Diagnoses and Interventions

> **Risk for injury to mother related to physiological processes of labor**

Nursing interventions

Help the woman maintain a comfortable position.

Encourage ambulation as tolerated if the membranes are unruptured and/or if the presenting part is well applied to cervix, to avoid prolapse of cord.

If membranes are ruptured and presenting part is not engaged, the woman should be maintained at bed rest in a comfortable position, avoiding supine hypotension.

Assess TPR and BP at least q4h.

Plot cervical dilation and fetal descent on a labor graph to assess the progress of the labor.

Offer clear liquids as ordered.

Encourage frequent voiding and help the woman to the bathroom as needed if presenting part is well applied to the cervix.

Measure intake and output.

Check urine for protein and glucose as indicated.

Initiate IV with isotonic solution (lactated Ringer's solution, normal saline) if ordered.

Prehydrate with 1000 to 1500 ml of fluid before regional anesthesia.

Maintain dosing of prelabor medications as ordered (anticonvulsants, antihypertensives, or methadone).

Expected outcome

The woman experiences no injury related to labor as evidenced by comfort, adequate hydration, absence of hypotensive episodes related to regional anesthesia, absence of distended bladder, and maintenance of prelabor medical status.

> **Pain and anxiety related to lack of information on physiological processes of labor**

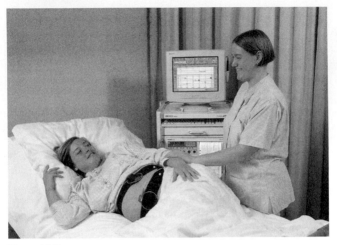

Figure 10-2
Externally monitored woman in the lateral position.
(Courtesy Philips Medical Systems, Böblingen, Germany.)

Nursing interventions

Nursing interventions during *active* labor

Maintain quiet and calm environment.

Avoid having persons in room who are not directly caring for the woman or providing support, to decrease anxiety.

Make sure nurse communication device is accessible.

Assist with position changes.

Encourage lateral position (Figure 10-2).

Assist with breathing/relaxation techniques.

Encourage significant other to be involved in support activities.

Apply cool compresses to forehead as needed.

Apply sacral pressure as needed during contractions to relieve discomfort.

Encourage support person to give back rub and to apply sacral pressure as needed.

Change gown and linens as needed.

Change pad under buttocks as needed.

Give pain medication as ordered.

Assist with administration of local or regional anesthetic.

Nursing interventions during *transitional* labor

    Palpate abdomen very lightly, and only as often as necessary if abdomen is hypersensitive.

    Prepare for vomiting episodes.

    Encourage the woman to empty bladder.

    Maintain warmth as necessary.

    Encourage the woman to avoid pushing until cervix completely dilated.

    Encourage use of panting or rapid-blowing breathing technique.

    Support laboring-down process.

    Provide reassurance that transition is relatively short compared with other phases of labor.

    Accept aggression or other coping behaviors and avoid negative comments.

    Focus on the woman and support her by using calm voice, touch, and positive reinforcement.

Expected outcome

The woman experiences manageable pain and minimal anxiety as evidenced by verbalization of same. She complies with assistive directions by staff. She has continuing interaction with significant other/family.

> **Risk for impaired oral mucous membranes related to mouth breathing**

Nursing interventions

Administer oral hygiene as needed between contractions.

Suck on ice chips, wet washcloths, or sour lollipops unless contraindicated.

Rinse mouth with water and/or mouthwash.

Apply petroleum jelly or antichapping lipsticks to dry lips as needed.

Expected outcome

The woman does not experience disruption in tissue layers of oral cavity.

> **Risk for ineffective tissue perfusion related to impaired transport of oxygen associated with uterine contractions and/or uteroplacental insufficiency**

Nursing interventions

Note frequency, duration, and strength of contractions according to facility protocols.

Evaluate and interpret FHR tracings.

Auscultate FHR:

> For 1 minute immediately after uterine contractions in nonelectronically monitored labor

> Every 15 to 30 minutes and as required by facility policy

> Assess FHR immediately after spontaneous or artificial amniotomy to assess for prolapsed umbilical cord.

Assess maternal vital signs per institutional protocol and as appropriate for risk factors.

Initiate intrauterine resuscitation protocols for nonreassuring fetal findings as indicated.

Turn the woman to the lateral position.

Discontinue oxytocin or uterotonic agent (prostaglandin).

Increase rate of isotonic IV solution.

Administer 100% oxygen by snug facemask at 8 to 10 L/min.

Notify physician of the situation.

Expected outcome

The woman gives birth to a newborn in good condition with Apgar score of 8 or higher at 5 minutes of age.

Education of the Woman and Family

Allay anxiety as much as possible by doing the following:

- Explain reasons for performing all procedures.
- Encourage spouse or significant other to remain with the woman to provide support during labor.
- Assist spouse or significant other in listening to fetal heart with fetoscope, Doppler, or ultrasound equipment.
- Provide supportive care that is respectful of the woman's and her family's knowledge of the labor process.
- Ask the woman if she wants additional support persons present for the labor and birth.
- Inform waiting family and friends about the woman's progress and inform the woman that they are waiting and interested.
- Reduce environmental stimuli that may contribute to anxiety and tension; provide a relaxed, restful atmosphere.

■ Reassure the woman at appropriate intervals that labor is progressing and that both the woman and fetus are doing well.

Care During Second and Third Stages of Labor

The second and third stages of labor consist of the expulsion of the fetus, placenta, and membranes after complete dilation of the cervix.

Assessment
Subjective data

Extreme anxiety
Patient stating, "Baby is coming"
Desire to defecate
Fear of losing control

Objective data

Involuntary bearing down/pushing
Grunting sounds
Vomiting
Involuntary shaking of thighs
Perspiration between nose and upper lip
Increase in bloody show
Prolonged second stage
Crowning

Potential complications

Nonreassuring FHR pattern
Difficult birth
    Cephalopelvic disproportion
    Shoulder dystocia
    Breech presentation
    Assisted delivery
        Forceps delivery
        Vacuum extraction
Vaginal laceration/extension of episiotomy
Cesarean birth
Infant bruising, fractures

Nursing Management
Care during delivery

Auscultate FHR every 5 minutes and/or after each push if electronic monitor is not used (if electronic monitor was used continuously during labor, then it should be continued in the delivery room until the time of delivery).

Evaluate FHR tracing every 5 minutes.

Pad stirrups or foot/leg supports if used.

Administer oxygen mask at 8 to 10 L/min as indicated.

Assist with breathing techniques:

Deep ventilation before and after each contraction.

Open-glottis breathing when pushing with contractions.

Observe perineum while pushing.

Notify midwife or physician if second stage is prolonged.

Prepare perineum according to hospital procedure.

Place nurse, spouse, and/or labor coach at head of delivery table to encourage the woman during delivery process.

Support laboring-down process.

Encourage long, sustained pushing rather than frequent short pushes; maintain open-glottis breathing.

Encourage the woman to push when she feels the urge to push.

Work with the woman to find a rhythm for pushing that is most effective for her.

Encourage complete relaxation between contractions.

Reassure the woman that she is doing well and is advancing the fetus with each push.

Apply cool, moist cloth to forehead as needed.

Keep suction catheter and meconium aspirator available and ready to use if meconium-stained amniotic fluid is present.

Plan for suctioning of naso-oropharynx after delivery of fetal head and before delivery of thorax to prevent meconium aspiration.

Have resuscitation equipment and neonatal resuscitation program (NRP)-trained personnel ready for delivery.

Assist in obtaining cord blood as indicated.

Assist physician or nurse-midwife as needed.

Immediate postpartum care ("fourth-stage" care)

Encourage the woman to inspect the infant as soon as possible.

Place the infant on the maternal abdomen to provide skin-to-skin contact if delivery room is warm.

Defer neonatal eye therapy for 1 to 2 hours after birth to promote eye contact with mother; administer eye therapy per hospital policy.

Assess maternal blood pressure and pulse per policy.

Add oxytocic drug as ordered to parenteral fluids.

Palpate fundus for tone several times in the first 2 hours after delivery (e.g., every 15 minutes for four times, then every 30 minutes for two times, or every 5 to 10 minutes for four times and as needed).

Massage fundus gently to promote contracting and to help prevent excessive blood loss.

Report signs of vaginal hemorrhage and flaccid noncontracted uterine fundus to health care provider stat.

Assess maternal blood pressure and pulse frequently during the first 2 hours after delivery (e.g., every 15 minutes for four times, then every 30 minutes for two times, or every 10 to 15 minutes for four times and as needed).

Administer perineal care before removing legs from stirrups to cleanse and inspect perineum.

Place sterile perineal pad under buttocks before transporting the woman to recovery area.

Place ice pack on episiotomy unless otherwise ordered to reduce swelling.

Maintain the woman's warmth with blankets as needed.

Place radiant heat warmer over upper part of the woman's bed or place dry newborn with warm blanket next to her so that she can visually inspect, touch, and/or breastfeed nude infant while preventing neonatal heat loss.

Encourage the woman and spouse and/or labor coach to be with the infant in delivery area, providing them with as much privacy as feasible, unless this is contraindicated by maternal or neonatal condition.

Encourage the mother to freely express her feelings about herself and her infant.

If the woman is apologetic for her behavior, explain that behaviors manifested in labor are normal and there is no reason to be embarrassed.

Documentation

Clear documentation related to fetal monitoring and care of the woman in labor contributes to a complete picture of the woman's labor. It is essential to have excellent records, especially because the information may be reviewed months or years later in legal action. The following information should be included:

1. Initiation of monitoring
   a. Patient's name and age
   b. Medical record number
   c. Date
   d. Midwife's or physician's name
   e. Time the monitor was attached and mode
   f. Testing/calibration
   g. Gravida _____; para _____
   h. Expected date of confinement (EDC)
   i. Risk factors (e.g., pregnancy-induced hypertension, diabetes)
   j. Membranes intact or ruptured
   k. Gestational age
   l. Dilation and station
2. During the course of monitoring
   a. Maternal position and repositioning in bed
   b. Vaginal examination and results
   c. Analgesia or anesthesia
   d. Medication/parenteral fluids
   e. Blood pressure, temperature, pulse, and respirations
   f. Voidings
   g. Oxygen given
   h. Emesis
   i. Pushing
   j. Fetal movement
   k. Any change in mode of monitoring
   l. Adjustments of equipment
      (1) Relocation of transducers
      (2) Type and adjustment of catheter
      (3) Replacement of electrode
      (4) Replacement or removal of IUPC/IUPT (intrauterine pressure catheter/transducer)
      (5) Flushing of IUPC/IUPT
   m. Identification of nonreassuring FHR patterns
   n. Interventions for nonreassuring FHR patterns
      (1) Repositioning
      (2) O_2 administration
      (3) Medications administered or discontinued

    (4) Increase in rate of IV

    (5) Amnioinfusion

    (6) Fetal pulse oximetry

The time of all aspects of care should be noted if the monitor does not automatically print the time. Evaluating the monitor strip at designated intervals ensures that someone has assessed the woman and the FHR on a regular basis and that any nonreassuring pattern has been identified and managed. The clarity and accuracy of documentation is important in identifying the cause of a specific FHR response to interventions, and for performance improvement and teaching purposes.

3. On completion of monitoring and delivery, the nurse should make the following summary notations:
   a. Delivery date and time
   b. Type of delivery
   c. Anesthesia
   d. Sex and weight of the infant
   e. Presentation
   f. Both 1- and 5-minute Apgar scores
   g. Maternal or neonatal complications
   h. Presence or absence of meconium; character of meconium if present
   i. Cord blood, if sample obtained

Documentation during the intrapartum and postpartum periods should include all routine aspects of assessment, diagnoses, interventions, and evaluation of patient care based on current standards of practice. Preprinted medical record forms for the perinatal woman are available from different companies, such as the Maternal/ Newborn Record System (Hollister, Libertyville, Ill.), and professional organizations, such as the American College of Obstetricians and Gynecologists (Washington, D.C.). To promote efficiency and consistency in documentation, a table or checklist format is used, which saves time but more importantly provides a comprehensive overview of the woman.

Computer-based documentation systems are available as well and provide archival and retrieval capabilities. They are usually available from the companies that manufacture fetal monitors, as well as from other companies such as the WatchChild system (Hill-Rom, Batesville Ind.) (Figure 10-3). With the advent of computer-based documentation systems, the process of documenting patient care across the perinatal continuum has become

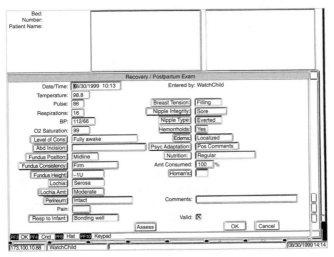

Figure 10-3
Monitor screen showing nursing documentation of routine assessment and postpartum care.
(Courtesy WatchChild, Hill-Rom Co., Inc., Batesville, Ind.)

streamlined and efficient. Multiple data entry points in the outpatient and inpatient setting, the combination of concurrent fetal surveillance and documentation, system interfaces with fetal and maternal monitors, and the ability to obtain statistical reports optimize the time spent and effectiveness of the perinatal nurse/midwife, the physician, and the managers who support the clinical service. Statistical information can be used to perform outcome studies and identify and monitor areas for improvement. In addition, this information can be used to meet the requirements of the state or province regulators and accrediting bodies. The benefits of a clear and complete record of a woman's care cannot be undervalued (Figure 10-4). Documentation systems, both paper based and computer based, are discussed from a risk-management perspective in Chapter 11.

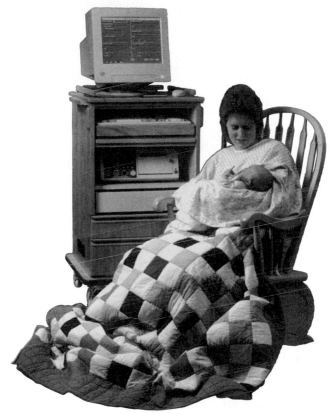

Figure 10-4
The desired outcome of quality patient care: a healthy post-partum mother and neonate.
(Courtesy WatchChild, Hill-Rom Co., Inc., Batesville, Ind.)

Risk Management 11

Risk management is the attempt to reduce the probability that a given risk will result in an adverse outcome (Rommal, 1996). Key components of a successful risk management program are avoiding preventable adverse outcomes and decreasing the risk of liability exposure (Simpson, Knox, 2000). When there is litigation related to an adverse neonatal or maternal outcome, the physician, midwife, hospital, and, often, individual perinatal nurses are named as defendants (Sinclair, 2000). Health care providers by nature and education want to help and care for people, so they are particularly devastated when they are sued by a client. They are likely to become preoccupied as unresolved lawsuits can take 3 or more years to be resolved (Queenan, 2001). The focus of this chapter is to provide some understanding of human error, to identify sources of potential errors during the perinatal period, to suggest strategies that may prevent or reduce errors, and to identify initial steps in the management of risks and actual errors.

Occurrence of Errors

The report "To Err Is Human: Building a Safer Health System," published by the Institute of Medicine (IOM; 2000) from its Committee on Quality of Health Care in America, brought national attention to statistics identifying medical errors as a significant cause of patient death or injury. Typical errors in health care settings relate to misunderstandings, erroneous use of medical devices, medication errors, lack of communication as patients move from one setting or one care provider to the next, unintended acts of omission such as not doing or responding to something, and acts of commission such as doing something outside the standard of care or practice. The IOM report advocated a shift from the old paradigm of "blame and train" when patient injuries occur, to identifying underlying system failures that have contributed to the preventable adverse outcome.

Through the efforts of the Joint Commission for the Accreditation of Healthcare Organizations (JCAHO), the National Association of Health Care Quality (NAHQ), and other organizations engaged in quality improvement in health care, patient safety has been established as the first priority in health care. The analysis of large numbers of injuries and reported errors confirms that adverse events most often result from error-prone systems and processes, not from error-prone individuals.

Human Error

Health care providers are educated and socialized to "do the right thing"—that is, to provide safe and appropriate care that results in a positive outcome. However, all health care providers are human, and humans make errors. Error is a normal part of the human experience and does not reflect laziness, bad intentions, or a personality defect (Reason, 2001). Understanding the nature of human errors (human factor analysis) is essential to any effort to prevent them. The most common types of human error are related to slips, trips, and lapses (Reason, 2001), which occur throughout a wide range of human activity. The following lists these activities in decreasing order of probability of occurrence (Park, 1997; Simpson, Knox 2003b):

- Stress (lack of time combined with high stakes—e.g., wrong sponge count in crash surgery)
- Change of shift (e.g., miscommunication)
- Inspection or monitoring (e.g., missing or not recognizing something)
- Arithmetic (e.g., miscalculating drug dosage)
- Omission (e.g., not doing or responding appropriately to something)
- Commission (doing something that is not consistent with an accepted standard of care)

Human errors are more likely to occur in the presence of personal and environmental factors known to increase the risk of error. Specific conditions have been identified that are known to increase the risk of error, and it is helpful to be aware of them. These conditions, listed in decreasing probability of risk of error, include the following (Reason, 2001; Simpson, Knox, 2003b).

1. Lack of familiarity with a task
2. Shortage of time

3. Poor communication
4. Information overload
5. Misperception of risk
6. Lack of experience (not necessarily training)
7. Poor instructions or procedures
8. Inadequate checking
9. Educational mismatch of a person with the task
10. Disturbed sleep pattern
11. Hostile environment
12. Monotony and boredom

Being aware of the most common types of errors and error-producing conditions helps in identifying, reducing, and managing risks in the perinatal setting. It is also helpful to understand human performance as it relates to knowledge, application of rules, and skills. For example, nurses function from a specialized knowledge base. As they become more skilled and experienced, they process information rapidly in recurrent activities and perform many duties automatically (Raines, 2000). *Skill-based performance* includes starting a routine IV, applying the external fetal monitor, and performing Leopold's maneuvers. Errors can occur when nurses' routines change or their attention is diverted, or from physiological (fatigue, illness), psychological (stress, family issues, frustration), or environmental (noise or unusual unit activity) factors.

Rule-based performance requires extra attention when an event differs from the routine. For example, when confronted with a commonly occurring problem, such as onset of fetal heart rate variable decelerations, experienced nurses operate from known and practiced rules or a series of learned responses for doing X when Y happens. When an unfamiliar problem arises, a rule-based error may occur because the wrong rule is chosen, the situation is not accurately perceived, or the rule is misapplied (Raines, 2000).

Knowledge-based performance requires controlled and conscious thought when nurses encounter a completely new, unfamiliar, or infrequently occurring situation. Examples of this type of situation are acute uterine rupture, development of a rarely seen sinusoidal fetal heart rate (FHR) pattern, unheralded prolonged FHR deceleration to 60 beats per minute or less, or maternal seizure in the absence of a known seizure-related condition. Errors can occur because of lack of information or data, or from misdirected attempts to match this novel situation to previous and more familiar situations. As the expertise of the nurse increases, the focus of control moves from a knowledge-based and rule-based performance to skill-based functions. What was once novel has become routine and the nurse does not usually have to resort to knowledge-based reasoning (Raines, 2000).

In summary, not all errors are preventable. And although humans do err, errors do not always result in injury or adverse outcomes, and not all adverse outcomes are the result of injury (Raines, 2000). It is unreasonable to presume that any one individual is the only person responsible for an error that results in injury to a patient. *It is inappropriate to rely on prevention of error as the sole means of creating patient safety.* Systems should be in place that will catch errors before they result in adverse outcomes; however, systems are subject to human and environmental variations. The role of risk management in the perinatal setting is twofold: to reduce the probability that a given risk will result in a poor outcome, and to recognize, mitigate, or minimize the consequences of the event rather than relying on prevention of error as the sole means of creating patient safety (Rommal, 1996; Simpson, Knox, 2000).

Common Errors in Perinatal Care

The most common errors leading to injury in perinatal care are as follows (Rommal, 1996; Knox et al, 1999; Simpson, Knox, 2000, 2003a,b):

- Lack of accurate interpretation of fetal monitoring, resulting in lack of timely recognition of both antepartum and intrapartum fetal compromise
- Lack of appropriate response to nonreassuring fetal heart rate tracings
- Delay in decision for, or initiation of, cesarean delivery as indicated by fetal or maternal status
- Lack of appropriate skills to perform neonatal resuscitation
- Nonindicated use for induction or augmentation of labor; failure to discontinue in presence of nonreassuring FHR pattern; excessive amount resulting in hyperactivity or uterine rupture
- Inappropriate use of forceps or vacuum extractor resulting in fetal trauma
- Application of fundal pressure
- Lack of communication between care providers (not done, not clear, not documented)
- Incomplete documentation

Prevention of Errors and Risk Reduction
High-Reliability Perinatal Units

Risk reduction and error prevention in perinatal care can be achieved when organizations direct their efforts to the avoidance of these common situations and the fostering of high-reliability characteristics. High reliability is described as the technical ability to operate technologically complex systems essentially without error over long periods. There are organizational characteristics and clinical practices that differentiate highly reliable perinatal units from those experiencing more error and injury. These organizations consider patient safety to be the first priority and have systems in place to prevent recognized sources of error and injury The primary characteristics of a high-reliability unit are as follows (Roberts, 1990a,b; Klein et al, 1995; Knox et al, 1999; Miller, 2003):

- The organization creates and fosters a safety-oriented culture.
- Decision making to enhance safety occurs at every level of the organization.
- Alarms can be called by anyone; hierarchy is minimized, rank is not an issue; anyone can challenge the status quo.
- Jobs are designed for safety; there is minimal reliance on memory; protocols, checklists, and forcing functions are built into the system.
- Teams that are expected to work together (e.g., physicians, midwives, and nurses participating in the same advanced fetal monitoring workshops) are trained and educated together.
- Multidisciplinary teams carry out drills for high-risk situations such as stat cesarean deliveries for fetal heart rate bradycardia or prolapsed umbilical cord.
- Communication is continuous, valued, and highly rewarded.
- The organization promotes the development of competencies and evaluates ongoing competence using a variety of learning techniques such as simulations, computer tutorials, and case studies in fetal monitoring.

Guidelines to Promote Safety and Reduce Risks

Recommendations and guidelines to promote patient safety and to decrease risk exposure include the following (Rommal, 1996; Simpson, Knox, 2000; AWHONN, 2003):

1. Policies, procedures, and protocols
   - Develop policies, procedures, and protocols based on accepted standards of care (Koniak-Griffin, 1999; McRae, 1999).

- Use nurse practice acts, standards promulgated by professional organizations (e.g., Association of Women's Health, Obstetric and Neonatal Nurses, American College of Obstetricians and Gynecologists, Society of Gynecologists and Obstetricians of Canada [SGOC]), journals, textbooks, and particularly evidence-based practice reports as sources for developing policies, procedures, and protocols (Mahlmeister, 1999).

2. Competency
   - Verify the nurse's qualifications at the time of hire to ensure that they meet the prerequisites of the institution.
   - Develop tools to evaluate performance related to specific skills, knowledge base of physiology and pathophysiology, and the standard of care to which the nurse is held accountable, based on the facility's rules (i.e., policies, procedures, and protocols) (McRae, 1999).
   - Promote and support certification of nurses in fetal monitoring (Reeves, 2001).

3. Fetal monitoring
   - Standardize fetal assessment and monitoring language throughout the institution, and clarify definitions for fetal well-being and assessment (NICHD, 1997; AAP, ACOG, 2002). Avoid using the terms *fetal distress* and *birth asphyxia* (ACOG, 1998).
   - Accurately monitor FHR and uterine activity; use instrumentation appropriately.
   - Identify and interpret electronic fetal monitoring data accurately (ACOG, 1995; AWHONN, 1998; Mahlmeister, 2000).
   - Recognize nonreassuring fetal status in a timely manner by evaluating FHR (AWHONN, 1998) according to standard frequency guidelines as described in Chapter 6.
   - Implement intrauterine resuscitation techniques (AWHONN, 1998) to ameliorate nonreassuring FHR tracings (e.g., maternal repositioning, increasing fluids, oxygen)
   - Communicate findings and efforts to correct nonreassuring FHR patterns to physician or midwife in a clear and unambiguous manner (Box 11-1).
   - Avoid removing the monitor in the presence of a nonreassuring pattern; continue fetal assessment until birth, including monitoring until the abdominal preparation is begun on women who are having a cesarean delivery (AAP, ACOG, 2002).

Box 11-1   Achieving Clear and Unambiguous Nurse-to-Physician Communication

1. Avoid ambiguity, hedging (e.g., "I'm concerned" or "I'm worried"), and confusion.
2. Be clear and direct in requests for orders and provider attendance at the bedside, and in the reason for the request.
3. Remember that your discussion is about the fetus.
   I am requesting that you come in now to evaluate this patient.
4. State facts. What do you see on the tracing? What have you done? What needs to be done?
   The baseline heart rate has increased from the 140s to the 160s and there are worsening variable decelerations. I have repositioned this patient, turned off the oxytocin, and given her a bolus of 500 ml of her primary IV, and she has oxygen at 10 L/min by mask. The fetal heart rate is not improving.
5. Be specific about what you are requesting.
   This patient needs further medical evaluation, and I am requesting that you come to the bedside now. It is 2:00 A.M. When can I expect you?
6. Restate the physician's response.
   I am confirming that you received my report and stated that you do not agree to come to the bedside now.
7. State what you will document.
   I am documenting in the patient record that I have requested that you come in now to evaluate this patient and her fetus, and that you decline to do so. Is there any change in your plan?
8. Ask for an alternative.
   Would you like me to call someone else to evaluate this patient in your absence? I will document your response to my question.
9. State what you will do now.
   Thank you. I will proceed to call Dr. X per your request.
   OR
   I will call Dr. X now and request that he/she come in to assess your patient and her fetus because your response time does not support safe care for this patient and her fetus.

4. Neonatal resuscitation
   - Ensure availability of appropriately trained and certified staff; redeploy staff as necessary to provide optimal care.
   - Prepare appropriate equipment and medications prior to delivery.

5. Organizational resources and systems to support timely interventions when FHR is nonreassuring
   - Have sufficient staff or be able to redeploy staff as needed. During the intrapartum period, the nurse-to-patient ratio should be 1:2 or 1:1, depending on the stage of labor and the complexity of the situation (AAP, ACOG, 2002; AWHONN, 2003). Staffing should be sufficient to begin a cesarean delivery within 30 minutes of a physician's decision to operate (AAP, ACOG, 2002). A more expeditious delivery (<30 minutes) may be necessary in cases of abruptio placentae, prolapse of the umbilical cord, hemorrhage secondary to placenta previa, and uterine rupture (AAP, ACOG, 2002).
   - Have systems in place that ensure a physician's timely response to the perinatal unit when needed and requested (e.g., in cases of a nonreassuring FHR pattern, uterine hyperstimulation with oxytocin with fetal intolerance to labor, vaginal birth after cesarean [VBAC] delivery). A policy that exists in high-reliability perinatal units is that "a physician will come to the unit when requested by a nurse" (Knox et al, 1999).

6. Perinatal teamwork: collaboration and respect
   - Recognize multidisciplinary teams as the unifying principle that creates operational excellence and success. "In any situation requiring a real-time combination of multiple skills, experiences and judgment, *teams,* as opposed to individuals, create superior performance" (Simpson, Knox, 2001, p. 56).
   - Engage in team building through a multidisciplinary clinical practice or performance improvement committee to come to consensus on both routine and problematic practices, to improve communication, to build trust and confidence in one another, and to achieve performance goals (Katzenback, Smith, 1993; Simpson, Knox, 2001).
   - Work toward creating a culture in which everyone feels free to ask for help (Veltman, 2003).

7. Interdisciplinary case reviews
   - Evaluate errors that were caught immediately (good catches) and events that could have had adverse consequences but did

not (near misses); view them as golden opportunities to strengthen systems that promote safety (Veltman, 2003). Do not wait for an issue to be identified on a quality improvement screen, as this indicates that an error that resulted in an adverse outcome did occur.

- Focus actions on the patient's well-being.
- Eliminate a blame-based environment.
- Focus reviews on the six most common allegations of obstetric malpractice claims (Veltman, 2003). These are as follows:
  (1) Failure to recognize or respond to nonreassuring fetal status
  (2) Failure to do a timely delivery
  (3) Failure to conduct proper resuscitation
  (4) Negligently causing vacuum or forceps injuries
  (5) Failure to prevent and manage shoulder dystocia
  (6) Improper use of oxytocin

8. Chain of command/communication issues
   - Develop a chain of command (Figure 11-1) with key medical, nursing, administrative, and risk-management leaders.
   - Implement the chain of command (see Figure 11-1) when nurse and physician disagree (e.g., about tracing interpretation or management of the patient), or when the physician does not respond (Greenwald, Mondor, 2003).
   - Report any incidence of provider behavior that does not support quality or safe patient care, that increases risk to the patient, or that could contribute to an adverse outcome, to the quality/performance improvement committee, regardless of fear of retaliation or retribution, which, if it occurs, should be reported as well. "When people fail to engage in respectful interactions, things can get dangerous" (Knox et al, 1999).

9. Joint nurse/provider education
   - To provide consistency of information and expectations, hold forums on skills (e.g., a stat cesarean delivery drill), on conducting patient conferences, on reviewing fetal monitor tracings, and on any other activities that involve multidisciplinary team members.

Management of Risks and Adverse Outcomes

It is well recognized that obstetrics is one of the most litigious areas of medicine (McRae, 1999; Greenwald, Mondor, 2003).

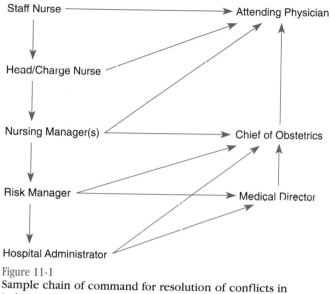

Figure 11-1
Sample chain of command for resolution of conflicts in judgment between nurse and health care provider.

When risk issues or an adverse outcome is identified, the woman's medical record is reviewed by the multidisciplinary health care team, which is responsible for analyzing risks and contributing factors that may have resulted in an adverse outcome. This cannot be done without adequate and appropriate documentation in the patient's medical record.

Documentation

Documentation in the woman's record is used to describe care and interventions provided in a sequential manner. This information may be stored or archived on an optical disk or other device (Figure 11-2). In some states, it is lawful to discard the paper strip once it is confirmed that all monitoring data is captured in the electronic system. Increasing evidence indicates that documentation should be done only once, on the paper labor flow sheet or in the electronic record, to avoid duplication (Kelly, 1999). Duplicative charting presents a significant risk of inconsistencies that can be questioned or challenged by plaintiff attorneys in the event of future litigation. Furthermore, duplicative documentation in the medical record and on the fetal monitor strip is unnecessarily labor intensive for nurses who are frequently fully occupied in care of the woman and fetus.

Record Storage and Retrieval

The fetal monitor tracing is a part of the patient's medical record; therefore storage, security, and record retrieval are the responsibility of the hospital's medical records department. If the paper strip is archived, each segment of the strip must be clearly identified per

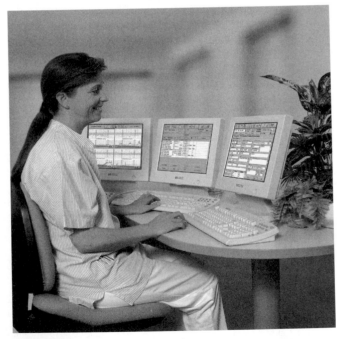

Figure 11-2
Data storage is an option with central monitoring systems. Information is stored on an optical disk and can be easily retrieved and printed in its original quality. A security system prevents the editing or addition of information to the stored data.
(Courtesy Philips Medical Systems, Böblingen, Germany.)

unit policy. The strips should be numbered sequentially and securely banded together for archiving. Confidentiality of the fetal monitor tracings must be maintained by storing them in a secure place until the woman's entire medical record is sent to the medical records department. A process must be in place to request and reliably retrieve all fetal monitoring tracings, whether on paper, microfilm, or electronic archival. In the event of litigation, any missing monitoring information makes a case difficult if not impossible to defend despite excellent care and complete compliance with established standards.

Elements of Malpractice

Failure to do something that a reasonable and prudent nurse would do in the same circumstances is known as malpractice or professional negligence. Nurses are held to national standards of care and practice within the "same or similar circumstances" and "reasonably expected" parameters. Inherent in this statement is the expectation that the nurse is knowledgeable about the standards of care and is fully competent to apply those standards when caring for patients (Mahlmeister, 2000).

Negligence is the failure to act in the required manner, causing harm to an individual. *Malpractice* is an unintentional act performed by a professional acting in a professional capacity, that causes harm to an individual. Under the rule *respondeat superior,* "let the master answer," an employer is held liable for acts of malpractice committed by an employee while performing duties for which she or he was hired.

For an action to fit the legal definition of malpractice, the following four elements must be met:

- *Duty:* The patient is owed a specific duty or standard of care.
- *Breach of duty:* There was a failure to meet the required standard of care.
- *Proximate cause:* A direct causal relationship exists between the breach of duty and the harm or injury to the patient.
- *Harm or injury:* Actual harm or injury occurred to the woman, fetus, or neonate as a result of the breach of duty.

Communication

When there is error, injury, or other adverse outcome, there should be written and well-understood procedures to guide staff. Notification of supervisory or management-level individuals should be timely, according to organizational policy. Appropriate quality assurance memos or incident reports should be completed for performance improvement purposes, but no reference to these items should be made in the medical record. The medical record should contain documentation of the facts surrounding the event and should be free from editorial commentary and potentially damaging, biased, or blaming comments.

When an adverse outcome occurs, the entire perinatal unit is usually aware of the event. There is great interest in finding out what happened, and the staff sincerely wants to support the team members involved by reviewing the event in detail. However, chart review and questions in the absence of a "need to know" must be avoided. Any discussions occurring outside an official quality improvement or risk management forum will be discoverable in the event of litigation and can be required to be repeated under oath. Perinatal care providers should be knowledgeable about the appropriate time and place to discuss events, and they should be compliant with the Health Insurance Portability and Accountability Act (HIPAA) regulations regarding protected patient information.

A critical incident debriefing by a skilled resource, such as an employee assistance program (EAP), a trained hospital-based team, a social worker, or a chaplain, provides an opportunity for staff to process feelings and concerns related to adverse outcomes and patient injuries in an environment free from discovery and blame. The critical incident debriefing is most effective when conducted as soon as possible after the occurrence of the event.

In the event of litigation, a plaintiff's attorney may attempt to make direct contact with nurses involved in the care of the allegedly injured patient. Hospital or unit orientation should include information about the correct response to such a request (refusal to discuss), and the requirement that the hospital's risk management department be notified and involved before any discussion with a plaintiff's attorney occurs.

Patient Disclosure

When an injury occurs, JCAHO standards require that information about how the error occurred and remedies available be disclosed to the woman and her family (JCAHO, 2003). During disclosure, the woman and her family should be informed that the factors involved in the injury will be investigated so that steps can be taken to reduce the likelihood of similar injury to other patients (National

Patient Safety Foundation, 2000). Disclosure should be made with the support of trained individuals; nurses should refrain from discussing the details of the event with the patient and family without appropriate support through the organization's disclosure process.

Reporting of Sentinel Events

Adverse events that meet the definition of a sentinel event (i.e., an unexpected occurrence involving death or serious physical or psychological injury, or the risk thereof) must be reported according to JCAHO and state department of health standards. A sentinel event signals the need for immediate investigation and response. The JCAHO specifically lists "any intrapartum maternal death and any perinatal death unrelated to a congenital condition in an infant with birthweight >2500 grams" as voluntarily reportable events (JCAHO, 2003). Following the report of a sentinel event, the organization must conduct a root-cause analysis and report the findings of that process to the JCAHO. The root-cause analysis identifies causal factors for the sentinel event and improvements in processes or systems that would decrease the likelihood of such events in the future. Root-cause analysis follows an event and focuses primarily on systems and processes, not individual performance.

Failure Mode, Effect, and Criticality Analysis

In June 2001, the JCAHO began requiring accredited hospitals to complete at least one yearly failure mode, effect, and criticality analysis (FMECA). An FMECA differs from a root-cause analysis in being a proactive, systematic examination of a process, such as fetal monitoring during labor, to identify ways in which failure *could* occur during the process. The assumption of the FMECA is that no matter how knowledgeable or careful people are, errors will occur and may even be *likely* to occur. Proactive identification of potential errors (failure modes) enables the organization to make changes in a process to prevent error and injury from occurring (JCAHO, 2003).

Summary

Risk management in perinatal care involves intentional action and process to avoid errors and to prevent injury or harm to mother and fetus. Risk management also involves response to errors and injury as required by the JCAHO, and management of litigation resulting from perinatal injury. System thinking about risk and error has replaced blame and focus on errors by individuals. There are specific perinatal risk reduction strategies related to use of fetal monitoring. An environment rich in competent care providers who practice as a team, speak the same language, avoid variances in practice, and have systems in place for timely clinical intervention supports the likelihood of that organization being one of high reliability.

References

American Academy of Pediatrics (AAP) and American College of Obstetricians and Gynecologists (ACOG): *Guidelines for perinatal care,* Washington, DC, 2002, The Academy and the College.

American College of Obstetricians and Gynecologists: Fetal heart rate patterns: Monitoring, interpretation, and managements, *Technical Bulletin* no. 207, Washington, DC, 1995, The College.

American College of Obstetricians and Gynecologists: Inappropriate use of the terms fetal distress and birth asphyxia, *Committee Opinion* no. 197, Washington, DC, 1998, The College.

Association of Women's Health, Obstetric and Neonatal Nurses (AWHONN): *Fetal heart monitoring: Principles and practices,* ed 3, Dubuque, Iowa, 2003, Kendall/Hunt.

Association of Women's Health, Obstetric and Neonatal Nurses: *Clinical competencies and education guide: Fetal surveillance in antepartum and intrapartum nursing practice,* ed 3, Washington, DC, 1998, The Association.

Institute of Medicine (IOM): *To err is human: Building a safer health system,* Washington, DC, 2000, National Academy Press.

Greenwald L, Mondor M: Malpractice and the perinatal nurse, *J Perinat Neonatal Nurs* 17(2):101-109, 2003.

Joint Commission on Accreditation of Healthcare Organizations (JCAHO): *Comprehensive manual for accreditation of hospitals,* Oak Brook, Ill., 2003, The Commission.

Katzenbach JR, Smith DK: *The wisdom of teams,* Boston, 1993, Harvard Business School Press.

Kelly CS: Perinatal computerized patient record and archiving systems: Pitfalls and enhancements for implementing a successful computerized medical record, *J Perinat Neonatal Nurs* 12(4):1-14, 1999.

Klein RL, Bigley JA, Roberts KH: Organization culture in high reliability organizations: An extension, *Human Relations* 48(1):1-23, 1995.

Knox G, Simpson K, Garite T: High Reliability Perinatal Units: An approach to the prevention of patient injury and medical malpractice claims, *J Healthcare Risk Manag* 19(2):24-32, 1999.

Koniak-Griffin D: Strategies for reducing the risk of malpractice litigation in perinatal nursing, *J Obstet Gynecol Neonatal Nurs* 28(3):291-299, 1999.

Mahlmeister L: Professional accountability and legal liability for the team leader and charge nurse, *J Obstet Gynecol Neonatal Nurs* 28(3):300-309, 1999.

Mahlmeister L: Legal implications of fetal heart assessment, *J Obstet Gynecol Neonatal Nurs* 2(5):517-526, 2000.

McRae M: Fetal surveillance and monitoring: Legal issues revisited, *J Obstet Gynecol Neonatal Nurs* 28(3):310-319, 1999.

Miller LA: Safety promotion and error reduction in perinatal care: Lesson from industry, *J Perinat Neonatal Nurs* 17(2):128-138, 2003.

National Institute of Child Health and Human Development (NICHD) Research Planning Workshop: Electronic fetal heart rate monitoring: Research guidelines for interpretation, *Am J Obstet Gynecol* 177(6): 1385-1390, 1997.

National Patient Safety Foundation (NPSF): *Talking to patients about health care injury: Statement of principle*, Chicago, 2000, The Foundation.

Park K: Human error. In Salvendy G, editor: *Handbook of human factors and ergonomics*, New York, 1997, Wiley.

Queenan JT: Professional liability: Storm warning, *Obstet Gyn* 98(2): 194-197, 2001.

Raines D: Making mistakes: Prevention is key to error-free health care, *AWHONN Lifelines* 4(1):35-39, 2000.

Reason JT: Understanding adverse events: The human factor. In Vincent C, editor: *Clinical risk management*, London, 2001, BMJ Books.

Reeves M: Building expertise: Making the case for fetal heart monitoring certification, *AWHONN Lifelines* 5(2):71-72, 2001.

Roberts KH: Some characteristics of high reliability organizations, *Organization Science* 1(2):160-177, 1990a.

Roberts KH: Managing hazardous organizations, *California Management Review* 32(summer):101-113, 1990b.

Rommal C: Risk management issues in the perinatal setting, *J Perinat Neonatal Nurs* 10(3):1-31, 1996.

Simpson KR, Knox GE: Risk management and EFM: Decreasing risk of adverse outcomes and liability exposure, *J Perinat Neonatal Nurs* 14(3):40-52, 2000.

Simpson KR, Knox GE: Perinatal teamwork, *AWHONN Lifelines* 5(5): 56-59, 2001.

Simpson KR, Knox GE: Common areas of litigation related to care during labor and birth: Recommendations to promote patient safety and decrease risk exposure, *J Perinat Neonatal Nurs* 17(2):94-109, 2003a.

Simpson KR, Knox GE: Adverse perinatal outcomes: Recognizing, understanding, and preventing common accidents, *AWHONN Lifelines* 7(3):224-235, 2003b.

Sinclair BP: Nurses and malpractice, *AWHONN Lifelines* 4(5):7, 2000.

Veltman L: Poor systems create liability for good providers. In Garza M, Piver JS: *Ob-Gyn Malpract Prevent* 10(7):49-56, 2003.

Appendix

Selected Pattern Interpretations at 1 cm/min Paper Speed

Cardiotocography (electronic fetal heart rate [FHR] monitoring) outside of North America is usually done at a paper speed of 1 cm/min, which is slower than the 3 cm/min paper speed used in North America. Note that the FHR range is from 50 to 210 beats per minute (bpm) and that each vertical line on the trace paper is 30 seconds of time (Figure A-1).

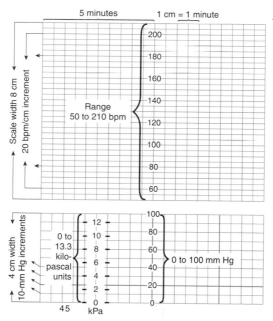

Figure A-1
Fetal monitor paper used in countries outside North America, with a paper speed of 1 cm/min.

Reactive Fetal Heart Rate on Admission

SIGNAL SOURCE	Spiral electrode and tocotransducer (1 cm/min)	
FHR	Baseline	120 to 130 bpm
	Variability	Moderate
	Periodic and episodic changes	Acceleration of FHR with uterine contractions and fetal movement
UTERINE ACTIVITY	Frequency	3½ to 4 minutes
	Duration	60 to 90 seconds

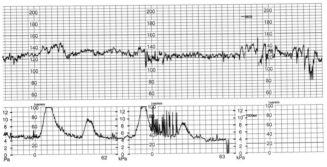

Figure A-2
1 cm/min
(Courtesy Dr. Lennart Nordström, Stockholm, Sweden.).

Reactive Nonstress Test

SIGNAL SOURCE   Ultrasound and tocotransducer (1 cm/min)

FHR   Baseline   135 to 140 bpm

Variability   Moderate

Episodic changes   Accelerations of FHR

Baseline rate shows a quiet period without accelerations and baseline variability of 5 to 10 bpm followed by an active period indicated by fetal movement profile (FMP) blocks. Note that there are more than two accelerations of >15 bpm lasting >15 seconds and an increase of variability.

UTERINE ACTIVITY   Not in active labor

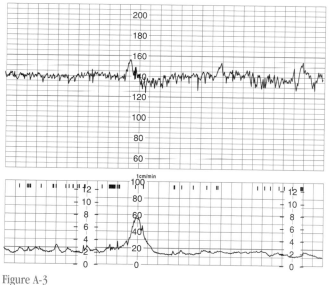

Figure A-3
1 cm/min
(Courtesy Philips Medical Systems, Böblingen, Germany.)

Normal Fetal Heart Rate Tracing

SIGNAL SOURCE	Spiral electrode and IUPT* (1 cm/min)	
FHR	Baseline	132 bpm
	Variability	Moderate
	Episodic changes	Accelerations of FHR
UTERINE ACTIVITY	Frequency	2 to 3 minutes
	Duration	60 seconds
	Intensity	58 mm Hg
	Resting tone	15 mm Hg

*Intrauterine pressure transducer (same as IUPC).

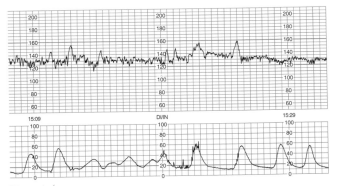

Figure A-4
1 cm/min
(Courtesy Dr. Herman P. van Geijn, Amsterdam, The Netherlands.)

Normal Trace of First Stage of Labor

SIGNAL SOURCE	Ultrasound and tocotransducer (1 cm/min)	
FHR	Baseline	100 to 110 bpm
	Variability	Moderate
	Episodic changes	Acceleration of FHR with fetal movement
UTERINE ACTIVITY	Frequency	3 to 4 minutes
	Duration	60 seconds

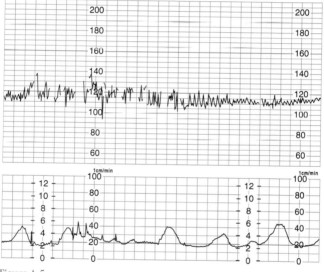

Figure A-5
1 cm/min
(Courtesy Philips Medical Systems, Böblingen, Germany.)

Uterine Hypertonia

SIGNAL SOURCE	Spiral electrode and IUPT (1 cm/min)	
FHR	Baseline	130 bpm
	Variability	Moderate
	Periodic changes	None
UTERINE ACTIVITY	Frequency	1 to 2 minutes
	Duration	60 seconds
	Intensity	50 to 60 mm Hg
	Resting tone	5 to 10 mm Hg

Note increase in resting tone with clustering of frequent uterine contractions.

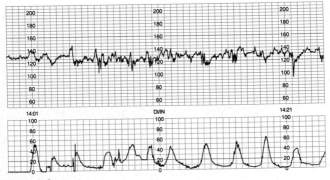

Figure A-6
1 cm/min
(Courtesy Dr. Herman P. van Geijn, Amsterdam, The Netherlands.)

Fluctuating Baseline/Variable Decelerations

SIGNAL SOURCE	Spiral electrode and tocotransducer (1 cm/min)	
FHR	Baseline	Fluctuating
	Variability	Moderate
	Episodic changes	Variable decelerations
UTERINE ACTIVITY	Frequency	3 to 3½ min
	Duration	60 to 90 seconds

This patient was a primigravida at 9 cm with a prolonged second stage. Fetal blood sampling revealed a pH of 7.25 and a lactate of 2.8 milliosmols/L (within normal limits).

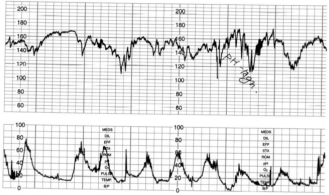

Figure A-7

1 cm/min

(Courtesy Dr. Lennart Nordström, Stockholm, Sweden.)

Sinusoidal Pattern

SIGNAL SOURCE	Ultrasound and tocotransducer (1 cm/min)
FHR	Baseline 180 bpm—tachycardia
	Variability Sinusoidal pattern
	Periodic/episodic None
	Fetus had severe anemia.
UTERINE ACTIVITY	Not in active labor; note the characteristic zigzag maternal respiratory movements on the uterine activity tracing.

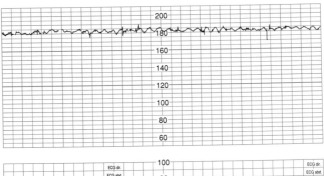

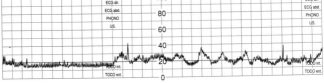

Figure A-8

1 cm/min

(Courtesy Philips Medical Systems, Böblingen, Germany.)

Tachycardia

SIGNAL SOURCE	Spiral electrode and IUPT (1 cm/min)	
FHR	Baseline	165 bpm
	Variability	Moderate
	Episodic changes	Accelerations and mild variable decelerations
UTERINE ACTIVITY	Frequency	1½ to 2 minutes
	Duration	60 seconds
	Intensity	Unable to determine exactly; approximately 40 to 50 mm Hg
	Resting tone	Unable to determine exactly; approximately 5 to 10 mm Hg

It does not appear that the UA was zeroed before use.

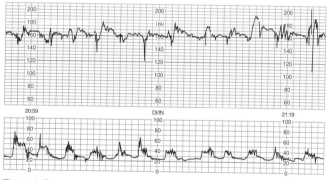

Figure A-9
1 cm/min
(Courtesy Dr. Herman P. van Geijn, Amsterdam, The Netherlands.)

Early Decelerations

SIGNAL SOURCE	Spiral electrode and tocotransducer (1 cm/min)	
FHR	Baseline	120 bpm
	Variability	Moderate
	Periodic changes	Early decelerations
UTERINE ACTIVITY	Frequency	4 to 5 minutes
	Duration	90 seconds

Note the mirror image of the early decelerations with the uterine contractions.

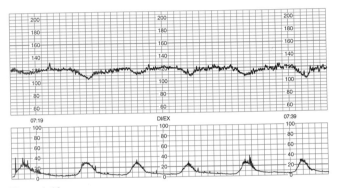

Figure A-10
1 cm/min
(Courtesy Dr. Herman P. van Geijn, Amsterdam, The Netherlands.)

Late Decelerations

SIGNAL SOURCE	Spiral electrode and IUPT (1 cm/min)	
FHR	Baseline	165 bpm
	Variability	Moderate
	Periodic changes	Repetitive late decelerations

Note that the nadir of the deceleration mirrors the amplitude of the uterine contraction.

UTERINE ACTIVITY	Frequency	2 to 4 minutes
	Duration	45 to 60 seconds
	Intensity	70 mm Hg
	Resting tone	15 mm Hg

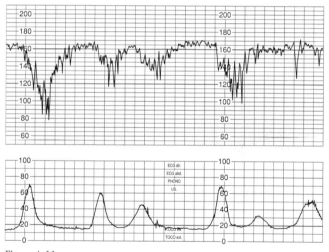

Figure A-11
1 cm/min
(Courtesy Philips Medical Systems, Böblingen, Germany.)

Mild Variable Decelerations

SIGNAL SOURCE	Spiral electrode and IUPT (1 cm/min)	
FHR	Baseline	135 to 140 bpm
	Variability	Moderate
	Episodic changes	Mild variable decelerations with shouldering and overshoot
UTERINE ACTIVITY	Frequency	2 minutes
	Duration	45 to 60 seconds
	Intensity	80 mm Hg
	Resting tone	5 to 10 mm Hg

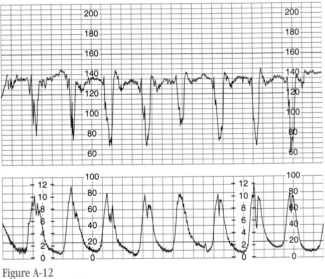

Figure A-12
1 cm/min
(Courtesy Philips Medical Systems, Böblingen, Germany.)

Variable Decelerations

SIGNAL SOURCE	Spiral electrode and IUPT (1 cm/min)	
FHR	Baseline	140 to 150 bpm
	Variability	Moderate
	Episodic changes	Mild to moderate variable decelerations; note shouldering
UTERINE ACTIVITY	Frequency	2 to 3 minutes
	Duration	60 to 90 seconds
	Intensity	60 to 80 mm Hg
	Resting tone	15 to 20 mm Hg

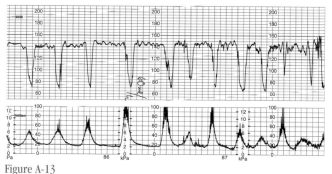

Figure A-13
1 cm/min
(Courtesy Dr. Lennart Nordström, Stockholm, Sweden.)

Variable Decelerations

SIGNAL SOURCE	Spiral electrode and tocotransducer (1 cm/min)	
FHR	Baseline	140 to 150 bpm
	Variability	Moderate
	Episodic changes	Variable decelerations with shouldering
UTERINE ACTIVITY	Frequency	2 to 3½ minutes
	Duration	60 to 90 seconds

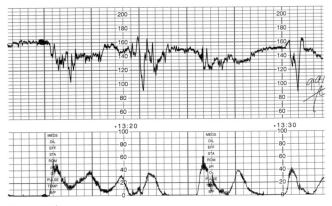

Figure A-14
1 cm/min
(Courtesy Dr. Lennart Nordström, Stockholm, Sweden.)

Moderate/Severe Variable Decelerations

SIGNAL SOURCE	Spiral electrode and tocotransducer (1 cm/min)	
FHR	Baseline	160 bpm (it was 140 bpm earlier in labor) progressing to unstable baseline FHR
	Variability	Moderate with episode of decreasing variability, slow return to baseline, and overshoot with some decelerations
	Episodic changes	Moderate to severe variable decelerations; note the shapes of the decelerations in the U, V, and W shapes characteristic of variable decelerations. Most of the decelerations last 60 seconds; the W-shaped decelerations, however, last appreciably longer.
UTERINE ACTIVITY	Frequency	2 to 4 minutes
	Duration	About 60 to 90 seconds

It is difficult to assess uterine activity in the first panel; this may be due to location of the tocotransducer and patient movement.

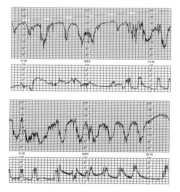

Figure A-15
1 cm/min
(Courtesy Dr. Herman P. van Geijn, Amsterdam, The Netherlands.)

Amnioinfusion for Variable Decelerations

SIGNAL SOURCE   Spiral electrode and IUPT (1 cm/min)

FHR   Baseline   Unstable initially, changing to 120 bpm after amnioinfusion

Variability   Moderate to marked (saltatory)

Episodic changes   Variable decelerations

Note the progression to a severe variable deceleration that was immediately relieved by the amnioinfusion bolus of 500 ml of fluid.

UTERINE ACTIVITY   Frequency   2 to 3 minutes

Duration   60 to 90 seconds

Intensity   60 mm Hg

Resting tone   20 mm Hg

It does not appear that the uterine activity baseline was zeroed before implementation of cardiotocography.

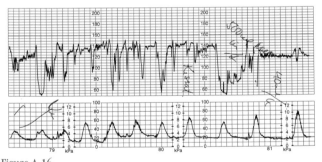

Figure A-16
1 cm/min
(Courtesy Dr. Lennart Nordström, Stockholm, Sweden.)

Prolonged Deceleration Secondary to Uterine Hyperstimulation

SIGNAL SOURCE	Spiral electrode and IUPT (1 cm/min)	
FHR	Baseline	140 bpm
	Variability	Moderate to marked
	Episodic changes	Prolonged deceleration below normal FHR range for 5 minutes
UTERINE ACTIVITY	Frequency	1½ to 2 minutes
	Duration	60 to 90 seconds
	Intensity	70 mm Hg
	Resting tone	20 mm Hg, increasing to 40 mm Hg before intervention

Oxytocin was discontinued immediately when hypertonus was observed but without effect on UA and FHR. A bolus of IV terbutaline (0.25 mg in 5 ml [indicated by the *arrow*]) relaxed the uterus within 2 minutes, and the FHR pattern returned to normal.

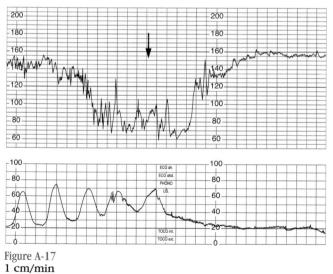

Figure A-17
1 cm/min
(Courtesy Philips Medical Systems, Böblingen, Germany.)

Glossary of Terms and Abbreviations

abruptio placentae   premature separation of the placenta before delivery of the fetus

acceleration   transient increase in the fetal heart rate (FHR)

acidemia   increased concentration of hydrogen ions in the blood

acidosis   a pathological condition marked by an increased concentration of hydrogen ions in tissue

ADT   admission, discharge, transfer

AFI   amniotic fluid index

amniocentesis   procedure in which amniotic fluid is removed from the uterine cavity by insertion of a needle through the abdominal and uterine walls into the amniotic sac

amnioinfusion   replacement of amniotic fluid with normal saline through an intrauterine pressure catheter

amnion   inner of the two fetal membranes forming the sac that encloses the fetus within the uterus

amniotomy   artificial rupture of the amniotic sac

anencephaly   absence of the cerebrum, cerebellum, and flat bones of the skull

angiography   x-ray examination of blood vessels made radiopaque by the injection of a radiopaque substance

anoxia   a total lack of oxygen in the tissue

ANS   autonomic nervous system

antepartum   occurring before birth

Apgar score   quantitative estimate of the condition of an infant at 1 and 5 minutes after birth, derived by assigning points to the quality of heart rate, respiratory effort, color, muscle tone, and response to stimulation; expressed as the sum of these points with the maximum, or best, score being 10

AROM   artificial rupture of membranes

artifact   irregularities on a fetal monitor tracing caused by electrical interference or poor reception of the FHR signal; may appear as scattered dots or lines

ASAP   as soon as possible

asphyxia condition in which there is hypoxia and metabolic acidosis

AST acoustic stimulation test; same as vibroacoustic stimulation test

AV atrioventricular

atelectasis collapse of the alveoli, or air sacs, of the lungs

augmentation correcting of ineffective uterine contractions (caused by dystocia) that occur after the start of spontaneous labor

baroceptor a pressure receptor; a nerve ending located in the walls of the carotid sinus and the aortic arch that is sensitive to stretching induced by changes in blood pressure

base deficit a measure of the amount of base buffer reserves below normal levels; insufficient base buffer to buffer acids; expressed as a positive number (e.g., 12 mEq/L); indicates metabolic acidosis

base excess a measure of the amount of base buffer reserves above normal levels; expressed as a negative number (e.g., −12 mEq/L); same as base deficit, but number is expressed as a negative number rather than as a positive number (i.e., base excess of −12 mEq/L is the same as base deficit of 12 mEq/L); indicates metabolic acidosis

baseline FHR range of FHR present between periodic changes over a 10-minute period

bilirubin pigment produced by the breakdown of hemoglobin in cell elements and in red blood cells

biparietal diameter distance from one parietal eminence to another; can be measured by ultrasound to determine gestational age

BL baseline (baseline FHR)

BP blood pressure

BPP biophysical profile

bpm beats per minute

bradycardia baseline FHR below 110 bpm for 10 minutes

cardiotography another term for electronic FHR monitoring

CBC complete blood count

CC cord compression

C/C/+1 used to indicate results of vaginal examination (e.g., cervix completely effaced/completely dilated/+1 station)

cephalopelvic disproportion (CPD) disparity between the size of the fetal head and the maternal pelvis, preventing vaginal delivery

cerebral palsy chronic static neuromuscular disability characterized by aberrant control of movement or posture, appearing early in life and not the result of recognized progressive disease

cervical ripening a complex process that culminates in the physical softening and distensibility of the cervix

chain of command a reporting mechanism to resolve conflicts that threaten the quality or safety of patient care

checkmark pattern a rare FHR pattern that resembles a checkmark ($\sqrt{}$ $\sqrt{}$ $\sqrt{}$ $\sqrt{}$ $\sqrt{}$); associated with fetal seizure activity

CIS clinical information system; networked computer technologies that process patient information including data collection, alerting, documentation, analysis, storage, and retrieval

chemoceptor sensory end organ capable of reacting to a chemical stimulus

chorion outer of the two membranes forming the sac that encloses the fetus within the uterus

chromosome a dark-stained body within the cell nucleus that carries hereditary factors (genes); there are 46 chromosomes in each cell except in the mature ovum and sperm, where that number is halved

circumvallate placenta placenta in which an overgrowth of the decidua separates the placental margin from the chorionic plate, producing a thick, white ring around the circumference of the placenta and a reduction in distribution of fetal blood vessels to the placental periphery

cm centimeter

CMV cytomegalovirus

CNS central nervous system

coupling two uterine contractions, one right after the other; the interval of time between the coupled contractions is less than the interval to the next uterine contraction or next set of coupled contractions

CP cerebral palsy

CRP C-reactive protein

CST contraction stress test

CT computed tomography

CTG cardiotocography; another term for electronic FHR monitoring

CVS chorionic villus sampling

d/c or D/C discontinue(d)

deceleration   a drop in the FHR; usually occurs in response to a uterine contraction

DFMC   daily fetal movement count

DIL   cervical dilatation

Doppler ultrasound   type of ultrasound that is reflected from moving interfaces, such as closure of fetal heart valves; Doppler ultrasound is used in electronic FHR monitors

DR   delivery room

DTR   deep tendon reflex

DW   dextrose in water

ECG   electrocardiogram

ED   early deceleration

EDC   expected date of confinement

EFF   effacement of the cervix

effleurage   gentle stroking of the abdomen; used during labor in the Lamaze method of prepared childbirth

EFM   electronic fetal monitor(ing)

epidural   area situated on or over the dura mater; regional anesthetic is often injected into the peridural (epidural) space of the spinal cord

episodic changes   spontaneous (nonperiodic) changes in the FHR that occur at any time and are not related to uterine contractions (e.g., accelerations and variable decelerations)

extraovular   outside the amniotic fluid space (between the chorionic membrane and the endometrial lining)

FAST   fetal acoustic stimulation test

FBM   fetal breathing movements

FECG   fetal electrocardiogram

FHM   fetal heart monitoring

FHR   fetal heart rate

FHT   fetal heart tones

FM   fetal movement

FMP   fetal movement profile

frequency (of contractions)   time from the onset of one uterine contraction to the onset of the next

FSpO$_2$ fetal oxygen saturation measured by fetal pulse oximetry

FT   fetal tone

GBS   group B streptococcus

gestation   pregnancy; the period of intrauterine fetal development from conception to birth

gestational age age of a conceptus computed from the first day of the last menstrual period to any point in time thereafter

gtt drops

HC head compression

HELLP syndrome a severe form of preeclampsia characterized by hemolysis (H), elevated liver enzymes (EL), and low platelets (LP)

HR heart rate

HUAM home uterine activity monitoring

hydramnios excessive volume of amniotic fluid, usually greater than 1.2 L; it is frequently seen in diabetic pregnancies and in fetuses with open neural tube defects (used interchangeably with polyhydramnios)

hydrocephaly increased accumulation of cerebrospinal fluid within the ventricles of the brain; may result from congenital anomalies, infection, injury, or brain tumor; the head is usually large and globular with a disproportionately small face; the increased head diameter is possible in the fetus and infant because the sutures of the skull have not closed

hydrostatic pressure pressure created in a fluid system

hyperstimulation of the uterus persistent pattern of tachysystole or single contractions lasting longer that 2 minutes, or uterine contractions of normal duration occurring within 1 minute of each other, resulting in demonstrated fetal intolerance to labor with evidence of nonreassuring FHR patterns

hyperthermia hyperpyrexia; high fever

hypertonic solution with a high osmotic pressure

hypertonus of the uterus excessive muscular tonus or tension; abnormally high uterine resting tone

hypothermia subnormal temperature of the body

hypotonic solution with a low osmotic pressure

hypoxemia decreased oxygen content in the blood

hypoxia a pathological condition marked by a decreased level of oxygen in tissue

hypoxic-ischemic encephalopathy a subtype of neonatal encephalopathy for which the etiology is considered to be limitation of oxygen and blood flow near the time of birth

IM intramuscular

induction stimulation of uterine contractions before the spontaneous onset of labor for the purpose of accomplishing delivery

infant mortality the number of deaths of infants under 1 year of age per 1000 live births in a given population per year

intervillous space space between the myometrium and placental villi that is filled with maternal blood

intrapartum occurring during labor or delivery

IUGR intrauterine growth restriction

IUP intrauterine pressure

IUPC intrauterine pressure catheter

IUPT intrauterine pressure transducer

IV intravenous (parenteral fluids)

IVP intravenous pyelogram

L liter

laboring down passive descent of the fetal head in the birth canal by uterine contractions (rather than active pushing) in the second stage of labor (after complete cervical dilatation), until the woman experiences a strong urge to push; benefits include decreased use of instrumental delivery, decrease in duration of second stage of labor, decreased maternal fatigue, decreased incidence of second- and third-degree lacerations and episiotomies

LAHF low-amplitude, high-frequency contractions

LATS long-acting thyroid-stimulating hormone

LD late deceleration

LDR labor/delivery/recovery room

L/S lecithin-to-sphingomyelin ratio

LTV long-term variability

macrosomia large body size as seen in some postmature infants and in those born to diabetic mothers

MECG maternal electrocardiogram

meconium pasty greenish mass that collects in the fetal intestine, usually expelled during the first 3 to 4 days after birth; its presence in amniotic fluid may be of concern, especially at the time of delivery should it be aspirated by the fetus; fetal naso-oropharynx is suctioned prior of delivery of the fetal body to avoid aspiration and resulting meconium aspiration syndrome

meningomyelocele protrusion of a portion of the spinal cord and membranes through a defect in the vertebral column

MHR maternal heart rate

min minutes

ml milliliter

mm Hg millimeters of mercury (unit of measure of pressure)

morbidity   the number of sick persons or cases of disease in relationship to a specific population

mortality   the death rate; the ratio of number of deaths to a given population

MRI   magnetic resonance imaging

MSpO$_2$ maternal oxygen saturation measured by pulse oximetry

mU   milliunits (used for oxytocin dosage, for example)

MVU   Montevideo units

MW   molecular weight

nadir   the lowest point of a curve; the depth or trough of a FHR deceleration

NBP   maternal noninvasive blood pressure

neonatal encephalopathy   a clinically defined syndrome of disturbed neurological function in the earliest days of life in the term infant, manifested by difficulty with initiating and maintaining respiration, depression of tone and reflexes, subnormal level of consciousness, and, often, seizures

nonperiodic   episodic or spontaneous changes in FHR that are not associated with uterine contractions, such as accelerations and variable decelerations

NRP   Neonatal Resuscitation Program

NS   normal saline

NST   non-stress test

nuchal   neck (as in umbilical cord around the fetal neck)

OCT   oxytocin challenge test

OD   optical density

osmolality   quantity of a solute existing in solution as molecules or ions or both; the concentration of a solution

osmotic pressure   pressure developed when two solutions of the same solute at different concentrations are separated by a membrane permeable to the solvent only

overshoot   transient acceleratory phase of the FHR that occurs at the end of some variable decelerations

P   pulse

PAC   premature atrial contraction

PAT   paroxysmal atrial tachycardia

PCB   paracervical block anesthesia

PDA   patent ductus arteriosus

PE   pelvic examination

peak   the highest point of a uterine contraction or FHR acceleration

periodic changes changes in the FHR that are associated with uterine contractions, such as early and late decelerations

PG phosphatidyl glycerol

PI phosphatidyl inositol

piezoelectric describes a substance that has the ability to convert energy from one form to another, such as mechanical pressure into electrical energy and vice versa, as with the ultrasound transducer

PIH pregnancy-induced hypertension

Pit Pitocin (oxytocin)

PL disaturated (acetone precipitated) lecithin

placenta previa placenta covering the internal cervical os

PMI point of maximal intensity

PO by mouth

polyhydramnios *see* hydramnios (terms used interchangeably)

prn as necessary

PROM premature rupture of membranes

PTL preterm labor

PVC premature ventricular contraction

q every

R respirations

RDS respiratory distress syndrome

reactivity fetus demonstrates episodes of FHR acceleration associated with fetal movement or stimuli; reactivity is associated with fetal well-being and forms the basis for the NST and VAS

resting tone intrauterine pressure between contractions (tonus)

R/O rule out; consider as a possibility

ROM rupture of membranes

SA sinoatrial

saltatory sudden abrupt changes in baseline FHR with marked, exaggerated, or excessive variability greater than 25 bpm

sawtooth an FHR pattern that resembles the teeth on a saw and is generally associated with arrhythmias

SE spiral electrode or scalp electrode

sec seconds

SGA small for gestational age

shouldering transient preacceleratory and postacceleratory phase of FHR at the beginning and end of some variable decelerations

sinusoidal HR pattern   baseline FHR that has a predominance of long-term variability with a characteristic sine wave pattern

spina bifida   congenital defect in the closure of the vertebral canal with a herniated protrusion of the meninges of the cord

spinal anesthesia   anesthesia produced by the injection of an anesthetic into the spinal subarachnoid space

Sub-Q   subcutaneous

SROM   spontaneous rupture of membranes

STA   station

STV   short-term variability

supine hypotension syndrome   weight and pressure of uterus on the ascending vena cava when the patient is in a supine position decreases venous return, cardiac output, and blood pressure

surfactant   phospholipid that normally lines the alveolar sacs after 34 weeks of gestation. Its presence prevents collapse (atelectasis) of the alveoli by permitting a small amount of air to remain in the alveoli on exhalation. The L/S ratio is a measure of the presence of surfactant in amniotic fluid. Neonates born without surfactant develop respiratory distress syndrome (RDS).

SVT   supraventricular tachycardia

T   temperature

tachycardia   baseline FHR above 160 bpm for 10 minutes

tachysystole   excessive uterine contraction frequency; six or more uterine contractions in consecutive 10-minute intervals (same as *hyperactivity of the uterus*)

tetany   state of increased neuromuscular irritability or spasm

toco   tocotransducer or tocodynamometer, an external device used to record uterine activity

tocodynamometer   pressure-sensing instrument for measuring the duration and frequency of uterine contractions (used interchangeably with tocotransducer)

tocolytics   drugs used to inhibit uterine contractions and stop labor

tocotransducer   *see* tocodynamometer (terms used interchangeably)

tonus   intrauterine pressure between contractions (resting tone)

transducer   device that converts energy from one form to another; sound or pressure can be converted into an electrical impulse and vice versa

trough   lowest point of a deceleration

UA   uterine activity

UC   uterine contraction

ultrasound transducer   instrument that uses high-frequency sound (ultrasound) to detect moving interfaces, such as the closure of fetal heart valves, to monitor the FHR

UPI   uteroplacental insufficiency

US   ultrasound

uterotonic   a pharmacological agent that increases the quality of muscle contraction of the uterus

UTI   urinary tract infection

variability   fluctuations in the baseline FHR

VAS   vibroacoustic stimulation

VBAC   vaginal birth after cesarean

VD   variable deceleration

VDRL   Venereal Disease Research Laboratories

VE   vaginal examination

Index

*Page numbers followed by b indicate
boxes; f, figures; t, tables.*